THE
GERIATRIC
SURVIVAL

H A N D B O O K

Barbara Acello, M.S., R.N.

A SKIDMORE-ROTH PUBLICATION

Cover Design: Barbara Barr, Visual Impact – Denver, CO

Typesetting: Barbara Barr, Visual Impact – Denver, CO

Developmental Editor: Wendy Thompson

Copy Editor: Maura McMillan

Notice: The author(s) and the publisher of this volume have taken care to make certain that all information is correct and compatible with the standards generally accepted at the time of publication.

Acello, Barbara
The Geriatric Survival Handbook
ISBN 1-56930-061-5
1. Nursing-Handbooks, manuals, etc. I. Skidmore-Roth, Linda.
II. Title
[DNLM: 1. Nursing Assessment-handbooks.
2. Nursing Process-handbooks. WY 39 G653n]
RT51.G66 1992
610.73-dc19
DNLM/DLC
for Library of Congress 89-5990 CIP
Skidmore-Roth Publishing, Inc.
2620 South Parker Road, #147
Aurora, Colorado 80014
(303) 306-1455
Web Address: http://www.skidmore-roth.com

TABLE OF CONTENTS

DRUG ADMINISTRATION

INFECTION CONTROL

TRANSCULTURAL NURSING

NURSING CONSIDERATIONS

NURSING CARE PLANNING

INTRODUCTION

INTRODUCTION

GERONTOLOGICAL NURSING PRACTICE

Gerontological nursing is focused on identification of the client's strengths, and assisting the client to use these strengths to maximize independence. The aging adult is involved in decision making to the fullest extent possible.

Factors the gerontological nurse must consider when caring for aging clients are:

- Consequences and complications of the aging process
- Individual effects of the aging process on each client; considering different rates at which people age
- Effect of losses on the client
- Social, economic, psychological, and biological factors
- Response of the client to the illness and treatment
- Cumulative effect of multiple chronic illnesses and degenerative processes
- The client's cultural values
- Societal attitudes and cultural values associated with aging

Basic Gerontological Nursing Practice

Basic gerontological nursing practice is performed in a number of settings. Responsibilities of the gerontological nurse including the delivery of direct care, management and development of non-professional caregivers, and evaluation of care and services for the client. All professional nurses caring for geriatric clients must have the basic knowledge and skills to do the following:

- Develop the care plan by using the nursing process
- Establish a therapeutic relationship with the client and family
- Recognize age related changes
- Collect data to determine health status and functional ability
- Function as a member of the interdisciplinary team
- Participate with clients, families, and other health care providers in making ethical decisions
- Act as an advocate for the aging client and family members
- Teach clients and families about measures that promote independence, maintain and restore health, and promote comfort

- Act as a source of referrals to other professionals or agencies, as appropriate
- Apply existing knowledge in geriatrics to nursing practice and interventions
- Protect the client's rights and autonomy
- Participate in continuing education, state and national professional organizations, and certification
- Apply the standards of gerontological nursing practice to improve clients' quality of care and quality of life.

STANDARDS OF CARE

The American Nurses Association sets practice standards for nursing. Measuring nursing care also evaluates accountability. The ANA *Scope and Standards of Gerontological Nursing Practice* provides a tool for which to measure accountability. Measurement criteria are listed for each standard so that nurses may assess their own performance and managers can assess staff members' performance.

The first standards were published in 1981. In 1994, the standards were revised to reflect the current scope of practice and address health promotion, health maintenance, disease prevention, and self care. The standards now address the full scope of gerontological nursing practice in two parts: Standards of Clinical Gerontological Nursing Care and Standards of Professional Gerontological Nursing Performance.

Standards of Clinical Gerontological Nursing Care

- Assessment
  Collection of client health data

- Diagnosis
  Analysis of assessment data to determine diagnosis

- Outcome Identification
  Identify outcomes individualized to the client

- Planning
  Developing a care plan that prescribes interventions necessary to attain expected outcomes

- Implementation
  Implementation of the interventions listed in the care plan

- Evaluation
  Evaluation of the client's progress toward attainment of expected outcomes

Standards of Professional
Gerontological Nursing Performance

Standards of professional performance describe a competent level of care, performance appraisal, education, collegiality, ethics, collaboration, research, and resource utilization. Gerontological nurses are expected to engage in appropriate activities for their level of education, position, and practice setting. Gerontological nurses should seek activities such as membership in professional organizations, specialty certification, further academic education, or advanced practice education.

- Quality of Care
  Evaluation of the effectiveness and the quality of nursing care

- Performance Appraisal
  Using applicable standards, statutes, and regulations to evaluate own nursing performance

- Education
  Maintaining knowledge of current nursing practices

- Collegiality
  Contributing to the professional growth of others by sharing information (clinical, research, etc.)

- Ethics
  Behaving ethically when making decisions and performing actions that affect clients

- Collaboration
  Involving others in the care of a client, including the family, the client, and other health care providers

- Reasearch
  Participating in and using research to improve the care of clients

- Resource Utilization
  Considers the safety, planning, cost, and effectiveness when participating in care of clients

DELEGATION

Delegation has become a major issue with the increasing use of unlicensed assistive personnel (UAP) in all health care settings. Delegation involves allowing an individual to perform a nursing activity. The licensed nurse is accountable for the performance and outcome of the nursing activity. It is in the nurse's best interest to ensure that the activity is delegated appropriately and that the UAP is able to perform the delegated nursing activity. Assessment should not be delegated. Although the UAP can gather data, such as vital signs, that contribute to an assessment, only a licensed professional nurse can assess a client.

The National Council of State Boards of Nursing formulated guidelines for delegation in 1996. Use of these guidelines ensures that the nurse is carrying out the delegation appropriately.

Appropriate delegation:

- Ensures that the UAP has received training and is competent to perform the nursing activity safely and effectively.

- Ensures that the licensed nurse can safely delegate the performance of the activity to a UAP because the client's care does not require frequent, repeated assessments during the delivery of the nursing activity.

- Ensures that the client's response to the performance of the delegated activity is reasonably predictable

- Is done because, in the professional opinion of the licensed nurse, the UAP will obtain the same or similar results as the licensed nurse in performing the nursing activity.

- Does not violate and is not prohibited by any law or rule.

Delegation of even simple nursing activities, such as checking blood pressure, is inappropriate in some situations. For example, the UAP may be qualified to check the blood pressure of a client during the admission process, but it may be inappropriate for the UAP to check the blood pressure of someone who is unstable or has had a critical procedure performed.

Not all nursing activities can be delegated. Many facilities use task lists for UAPs, giving the impression that the UAP can perform all of the listed duties at any time on any client. These lists create a false sense of competency. Nurse-directed delegation protects the client's safety.

The Five Rights of Delegation

- Right Task — one that can safely be delegated to the UAP for a specific client.

- Right Circumstances — appropriate setting, available resources and consideration of other relevant factors.

- Right Person — the proper person is delegating the right task to the right UAP for the right client.

- Right Direction/Communication — the UAP is given a clear, concise description of the nursing activity, including objectives, limits and expectations.

- Right Supervision — The UAP is appropriately monitored and evaluated. The licensed nurse intervenes, if necessary, and provides feedback to the UAP.

DEVELOPMENTAL TASKS OF AGING

- Retirement and adjustment to loss of work on identity, status, roles

- Retirement and adjustment to loss of income
- Declining physical function and adjustment to change in body image.
- Shift in roles and responsibilities with adult children, who may become the caretakers of parents in declining health.
- Realization of own mortality.
- Coping with death and loss of spouse, children, and friends.
- Coping with loss of social contacts due to death, physical inability, and relocation.
- Coping with social prejudices against ageism
- Life review and reminiscence.

AGING CHANGES

Integumentary System

Subcutaneous fat and elastin diminishes
- Skin thins, loses elasticity

Glandular activity decreases
- Skin dries, may become pruritic

Perspiration decreases
- Impaired temperature regulation

Reduced capillary blood flow
- Slower wound healing

Vascular fragility

- Senile purpura, increased skin tears

Reduced blood supply to lower extremities

Sensitivity to pressure and temperature decreases

Melanin production is decreased

- Loss of color in hair

Females develop facial and upper lip hair

Scalp, pubic, and axillary hair thins

Finger and toe nail growth slows

- Nails become brittle and develop longitudinal ridges

Musculoskeletal System

Elasticity and muscle mass diminishes

- Decreased strength and endurance, reaction time, and coordination

Bone demineralization

- Skeletal instability and shrinkage of intervertebral disks; less flexibility of spine and spinal curvature

Degenerative joint changes

- Limited range of motion, stiffness, pain

Cardiovascular System

Decline in cardiac output and recovery time

- Increased time for heart rate to return to normal following exercise

Slowing of heart rate

- Pulse slows, circulation less efficient

Blood perfusion to all organs decreases; brain receives more blood than other organs

Decreased elasticity of arteries; increased peripheral resistance

- Increased blood pressure

Dilation of veins

- Superficial blood vessels more prominent

Respiratory System

Muscular rigidity

- Decreased lung capacity and increased residual capacity

Cough less effective

- Increased pooling of secretions; increased risk of infection

Decreased functional capacity

- Dyspnea on exertion

Alveoli thicken

- Less effective gas exchange in lungs

Gastrointestinal System

Enamel of teeth thins

Increased incidence of periodontal disease

Decreased saliva production

Taste buds decrease, beginning with sweet and salt

Gag reflex less effective

- Increased risk of choking

Esophageal peristalsis slows; esophageal sphincter less effective

- Delayed entry of food into stomach; increased risk of aspiration

Gastric emptying delayed

- Food remains in stomach longer

Peristalsis and nerve sensation slows in large intestine

- Increasing incidence of constipation

Liver size decreases (over age 70)

Liver enzymes decrease

- Detoxification and drug metabolism slowed

Gallbladder empties less efficiently; bile thickens, cholesterol content increased

- Increased incidence of gallstones

Urinary System

Nephrons decrease
- Decreased filtration; decrease in excretory and reabsorptive function of tubules

Rate of glomerular filtration decreases
- Decreased clearance of drugs

BUN increases

Ability to conserve sodium diminishes

Bladder capacity decreases
- Increased frequency of urination

Renal function increases when lying down at rest
- Increased nocturia

Weakened bladder and perineal muscles
- Inadequate emptying of bladder; urine residual results in increased risk of infection
- Increased stress incontinence

Enlarged prostate
- Frequency, dribbling, obstruction in males; urine residual results in increased risk of infection

Neurological System

Neurons decrease in brain
- Decreased neurotransmitters; reduced synaptic transmission

Decreased cerebral blood flow and reduced oxygenation
- Takes additional time for motor and sensory tasks involving speed, balance, coordination, fine motor activities

Deep tendon reflexes decreased

Lens in eye less pliable
- Presbyopia, decreased accommodation; alteration in lens causes increased incidence of cataracts

Lens in eye yellows
- Distorted color perception

Accommodation of pupil size decreases
- Requires additional time to adjust to lighting changes

Consistency of vitreous humor changes
- Blurred vision

Decreased secretion of lacrimal glands
- Dryness, itching of eyes

Neurons in ears decrease; blood supply diminishes. Tissue in cochlea deteriorates; ossicles degenerate
- Reduced ability to hear; loss of tone discrimination; loss of ability to hear high frequency sounds occurs first

Taste buds decrease

- Decreased sensitivity for taste; causes increased condiment use

Less ability to discriminate pressure and temperature; diminished pain sensation

Diminished proprioception

- Difficulties with balance and coordination

Immune System

Autoantibodies increase

- Increased incidence of autoimmune disorders

Endocrine System

Delayed release of insulin by beta cells

- Increased blood sugar

Lower basal metabolism rate

Reproductive System-Women

Decreased estrogen production; menopause

- Decreased size of ovaries, uterus
- Vagina shortens, narrows, secretions become more alkaline and decrease
- Breast tissue decreases. Supporting musculature weakens

Reproductive System-Men

Testosterone production decreases

- Decreased size of testicles; sperm count decreases
- More time required for erection

Effect of Changes on Functional Status

Visual and auditory loss

- Apathy, mental confusion, disorientation, dependency, loss of control, loss of self care ability.

Change of environment

- Confusion, dependency, change in behavior and/or self esteem related to loss of control, relocation stress, possible sleep disturbances

Acute illness

- Dependence, change in behavior and/or self esteem related to loss of control, sleep disturbance, mental confusion

ASSESSMENT

ASSESSMENT

GERIATRIC ASSESSMENT COMPONENTS

The health assessment is a fluid, ongoing process in the geriatric client. Although assessment is the first step in the nursing process, it is not forgotten once completed. Geriatric assessment involves using observations and information to gather new data, recognize changes, and analyze needs.

Client profile

Name

Address

Telephone number

Race

Gender

Religion

Date of Birth

Language(s) spoken

Name of spouse or contact person

Family profile

Name and address of spouse

   -Date and cause of death, if deceased

Names and ages of children

Relationship with family members

Occupational profile

Type of work

Length of employment

Working hours

Home profile

Type of housing

-Owns or rents?

Number of levels

-Number of stairs

Location of bathroom

-Relationship of location of bathroom to
bedroom and living areas

Nearest neighbor

Availability of telephone

Type of community

Safety hazards

Ability of client to care for home

Presence of pets

Economic profile

Source of income

Is client receiving all available benefits?

Sources of financial concerns

Health insurance

Type and policy number

Health and social service providers

Physicians

Social workers

Visiting nurses

Public health agencies

Clinics

Hospitals

Community services

-Meal services

Social and leisure activities

Hobbies

Interests

Religious or spiritual profile

Spiritual belief system

Participation in religious activities

Health history

Family history

-Stroke

-Heart disease

- -Cancer
- -Diabetes
- -Hypertension
- -Tuberculosis

Previous health history

- -Hospitalizations
- -Surgeries
- -Fractures
- -Allergies
- -Drug sensitivities

Current health status

Current health problems

- -Client's understanding of problems
- -Limitations in functioning
- -Inability to perform ADL's
- -Appliances or prosthesis used

Client's main concerns in relation to health status

Family concerns

Medication profile

Review all medications (prescription and over the counter), vitamins, and herbs. For each medication, review:

- -Reason for drug

-How and where the drug was obtained

-Dosage

-Review of drug interactions

-Drug effectiveness

-Drug monitoring, serum levels and other factors

-Side effects

-Adverse reactions

-Evaluate continued need for drug

Emotional Status

-Affect

Cognitive Status

Verbal responsiveness

General nutritional status

Vital Signs

Height

Weight

Physical assessment

PHYSICAL ASSESSMENT MODIFICATIONS

Conducting a physical examination in the elderly can present many challenges. The examination may need to be adapted to account for sensory changes, slower response time, acute or chronic disease, and the client's need for assistance. Avoid making assumptions about the client's mental status or physical ability. Individualize the examination to accommodate the client's deficits. Anticipate that the exam may take longer than it would with a younger client. If a caregiver or family member is present, allow the client to state his or her wishes regarding whether this person will remain in the room during the examination.

Environmental Modification

- The elderly are particularly modest; arrange for a warm, private area
- Provide draping for comfort and warmth
- Bright non-glare lighting
- Eliminate background noise
- Warm instruments before touching client
- Provide pillows, props, or other positioning aids as needed
- Non-slip floor coverings
- Chairs with arms and high seats

Examining the Cognitively Impaired Client

- The client may be more comfortable if the caregiver is present; honor the client's choice.

- The client may need assistance dressing and undressing. However, allow the client to be as independent as possible. Observing how much can be done independently provides useful information about the client's abilities and degree of cognitive impairment.

- Approach the client in a warm, assuring manner and recognize him/her by name. Be patient. Cognitively impaired adults are sensitive to the moods of others and may discern if you are impatient or irritated.

- Speak in simple, concise terms. Give simple directions one step at a time; the cognitively impaired client may be unable to understand complex directions.

- Provide reassurance. Respond to the client's emotions. For example, if the client becomes fearful and starts to cry for her mother, reassure her that you understand how she feels and you will do everything you can to make her comfortable. Avoid reminding her that her mother is dead.

- Treat the cognitively impaired client with consideration and respect throughout the examination.
- Interview a collateral source separately to confirm and gather information

GERIATRIC HISTORY AND SYSTEMS ASSESSMENT

General

Age

Sex

Race

General health

Appearance

Nutritional status

   – Change in appetite

Chronic diseases

Fatigue

Fever

Night sweats

Sleeping problems

Height

Weight

Emotional status/affect

Verbal responsiveness

Vital Signs

Temperature

Pulse

- Carotid
- Apical
- Brachial
- Radial
- Femoral
- Popliteal
- Posterior tibialis
- Dorsalis pedis

Respirations

- Rate
- Depth
- Regularity
- Mouth/nasal

Blood Pressure

- Sitting
- Supine
- Standing
- Right arm
- Left arm

Respiratory System

Dates of last:
- – Tuberculin test
- – Chest x-ray
- – Influenza vaccine
- – Pneumococcal vaccine

Breath Sounds
- – Pitch
- – Quality
- – Intensity
- – Duration
- – Normal
- – Adventitious

Cough
- – Productive
- – Non-productive

Hemoptysis

Dyspnea

Orthopnea

Breath odor
- – Fruity
- – Alcohol
- – Ammonia
- – Clover
- – Foul

ASSESSMENT

Chest

Symmetry

Expansion

Scars

Structural abnormalities

Anteroposterior and lateral chest diameter

Crepitus

Pain/Sensitivity

Palpable masses

Tactile fremitus

Sinus

- Pain

- Infection

- Drainage

Nares/Sinuses

- Patency

- Lesions

- Masses

Epistaxis

Obstruction

Pain

Deviated septum

Rhinorrhea

Postnasal drip

Ability to differentiate common scents

Cardiovascular System

Mental status

Generalized color

Energy level

History of dizziness, edema, palpitations, blackouts

Chest pain

Shortness of breath

Neck vein distention

Cardiac Patterns

- Rate
- Rhythm
- PMI
- Thrills
- Murmurs
- Jugular venous pressure
- Palpitations
- ECG (or date of last ECG)

Carotid pulses

- Bruits

Pacemaker

Vessels

- Carotid
- Jugular

- Strength of pulses
- Symmetry of pulses
- Bruits
- Capillary refill
- Varicosities
- Thrombophlebitis

Condition of nails

Presence of hair on extremities

Lymph nodes

- Shape
- Mobility
- Tenderness
- Enlargement

Integumentary System

Skin color

- Pink/normal color for race
- Pale
- Ruddy
- Erythema
- Jaundice
- Cyanosis
- Mottled
- Blanched

Vascularity
- Bleeding
- Ecchymosis
- Petechiae
- Senile purpura

Edema
1+ =slight pitting, normal contour
2+ =deeper pitting, contours present
3+ =deep pitting, appearance puffy
4+ =deep pitting, frankly swollen

Skin temperature

Skin turgor

Texture
- Pruritis
- Dryness
- Scars

Nevi changes

Rash, lesions
- Type
- Size
- Color
- Shape
- Distribution

Masses

- Location
- Shape
- Size
- Tenderness
- Mobility

Nails

- Texture
- Color
- Lines
- Nail changes

Hair

- Distribution
- Hair loss
- Amount
- Consistency
- Color
- Texture

Scalp

- Itching
- Soreness
- Lesions
- Redness
- Sensitivity

Corns

Bunions

Calluses

Neurological System

Level of Consciousness

- Alert, oriented

- Lethargic

- Obtunded

- Stuporous

- Semicomatose

- Comatose

Head

- Pain

- Lesions

- Edema

Face

- Symmetry

- Expression

- Color

- Scars

- Rashes

- Lesions

- Facial pain

- Numbness

Eyes

- Appearance of eyelids
- Acuity
- Change in visual capacity
- Glasses
- Contacts
- Prosthesis
- Amblyopia
- Photophobia
- Diplopia
- Extraocular movements
- Pain
- Cataracts
- Glaucoma
- Pruritis
- Redness
- Drainage
- Ptosis
- Conjunctiva
- Sclera
- Vascularity

Pupils

- Size
- Shape
- PERRLA

Neck

- Symmetry
- Active Range of Motion
- Passive Range of Motion
- Pain
- Stiffness

Extremities

- Tingling
- Edema
- Stiffness
- Pain

Reflexes

- Deep tendon reflexes
- Biceps
- Triceps
- Patellar
- Babinski
- Achilles tendon

Superficial reflexes

- Pharyngeal
- Abdominal
- Plantar

Grading reflexes

- 0=No response
- 1+=Diminished
- 2+=Normal
- 3+=Brisk
- 4+=Hyperactive

Ears

- Loss of hearing/hearing aid
- Hearing capacity/ability to hear watch tick
- Pain
- Itching
- Discharge
- Infections
- Tinnitus
- Vertigo
- Wax deposits

History of seizures

Voice

- Tone
- Quality
- Articulation
- Speech pattern

Gastrointestinal System

   Appetite

   Diet

   Swallowing

   Pain

   Indigestion

   Regurgitation

   Nausea

   Vomiting

   Mouth/throat

   Color

   Odor

   Pain

   Speech/hoarseness

   Swallowing

   Chewing

   Taste

   Ulcerations

   Lesions

   Altered taste

Teeth/gums

- Date of last dental exam
- Caries
- Difficulty chewing

Dentures

- Examine fit and condition
- Remove dentures, inspect and palpate gums (with gloved hand)

Bleeding

Gag reflex

Abdomen

Size/contour

Symmetry

Dilated vessels

Muscle tone/adipose tissue

Rashes

Scars/Striae

Fluid/ascites

Distention/rigidity

- Auscultate RUQ, RLQ, LUQ, LLQ
  - Hypoactive
  - Hyperactive
- Auscultate liver/spleen for friction rubs

- Percuss
- Palpate
  - Pain/guarding

Rectum

- Masses
- Bleeding
- Hemorrhoids
- Fissures
- Excoriation/lesions
- Rash/itching
- Abcess
- Burning/pain

Bowel Elimination

- Normal pattern
- Constipation
- Diarrhea
- Flatus
- Laxative use

Renal System

Urinary Output

- Amount
- Color
- Odor

- Frequency
- Urgency
- Hesitancy
- Burning
- Pain
- Dribbling
- Nocturia
- Hematuria
- Oliguria
- Polyuria

Bladder Distention

Flank pain

History of incontinence

Daily Fluid Intake

- Water
- Alcohol
- Soft drinks
- Caffeine

Musculoskeletal System

Level of Activity

Gait

Prosthesis

Extremities
- Size/shape
- Symmetry
- Color
- Warmth
- Range of Motion
- Scars
- Bruises
- Rash
- Ulcerations
- Numbness
- Tingling
- Edema
- Prosthesis
- Fracture
- Infection/bone
- Intermittent claudication

Joints
- Range of Motion
- Deformities
- Stiffness
- Edema
- Pain

Muscles

- Conditioning/tone
- Spasms
- Tremors
- Strength/weakness

Back

- Pain
- Spinal abnormalities
- Kyphosis
- Scoliosis
- Lordosis

Reproductive System

History of venereal disease

Female

- History of pregnancies
- Menstrual pattern
- Gynecological problems
- Date of last pap smear/gynecological exam
- Dyspareunia
- Post-coital bleeding
- Inflammation
- Irritation
- Discharge

- Prolapse
- Edema
- Ulceration
- Nodules
- Masses
- Pain/tenderness

Breasts

- Date of last mammogram
- Last breast exam
- Client's knowledge of breast self-examination
- Breast changes
- Discharge
- Contour
- Symmetry
- Inflammation
- Scars
- Masses
  - Location
  - Size
  - Mobility
  - Pain/tenderness
  - Nipple discharge
  - Nipple inversion
  - Ulcerations

Axillae
- Nodes
- Enlargement
- Tenderness
- Rash

Male

Date of last prostate examination

Penis
- Discharge
- Lesions
- Foreskin
- Pain

Scrotum
- Edema
- Nodules
- Lesions
- Tenderness

Testes
- Edema
- Masses

Prostate
- Masses
- Tenderness

Breasts
- Nipples
- Pain
- Changes in breasts

Endocrine System

Previous diagnosis

Heat intolerance

Cold intolerance

Exopthalamos

Goiter

Skin pigmentation/texture changes

Hair changes

Hormone therapy

Polydipsia

Polyuria

Polyphagia

Central Nervous System

Previous diagnosis

Headaches

Seizures

Syncope

Paralysis

Paresis

Paresthesias

Coordination problems

Tic/tremor/spasms

Loss of consciousness

Behavior changes

Nervousness

Sensory problems

Cognitive ability

Head injury

Memory

- Recent
- Present
- Remote

Psychosocial

Anxiety

Depression

Insomnia

Crying spells

Nervous

Fearful

Difficulty making decisions

Difficulty concentrating

SEQUENCE OF PHYSICAL ASSESSMENT

1. Wash hands.
2. Assemble equipment.
3. Provide privacy.
4. Approach client with a sincere, caring attitude.
5. Make eye contact, call client by proper name, introduce self.
6. Obtain height, weight, vital signs.
7. Obtain history.
8. Explain each assessment procedure.
9. Perform system assessment.
10. Check hair and scalp for hair loss, lesions, rashes.
11. Check facial expression or unusual movements.
12. Check pupils.
13. Check corneal blink reflex and visual acuity.
14. Test function of trigeminal nerve.
15. Inspect ears.
16. Check nose, mouth, teeth, and gag reflex.
17. Note active and passive range of motion of neck.
18. Palpate neck, check lymph nodes.
19. Palpate thyroid.
20. Palpate carotid pulse.

21. Check for venous distention.

22. Inspect chest symmetry.

23. Determine pattern of respiration.

24. Inspect spine.

25. Auscultate posterior lung fields.

26. Inspect anterior chest, breasts, and axilla.

27. Auscultate and percuss anterior lung fields.

28. Inspect hands and arms.

29. Check shoulder, arm, elbow, wrist range of motion.

30. Auscultate heart sounds.

31. Ask client to assume supine position.

32. Inspect, auscultate, palpate, and percuss abdomen and flanks.

33. Percuss liver.

34. Inspect inguinal area.

35. Palpate and auscultate femoral arteries.

36. Check range of motion and muscular strength in hips, knees, ankles.

37. Palpate popliteal and pedal pulses.

38. Inspect and palpate genitalia.

39. Check deep tendon reflexes and Babinski's sign.

THE KATZ INDEX OF ACTIVITIES OF DAILY LIVING

The Katz Index of Activities of Daily Living is frequently used in geriatric clients to determine functional ability. The tool can also be used to assess improvement or deterioration. Use of the tool is based on the client's actual status, not ability. Hence, if a client refuses to perform a function, "he or she is considered to be not performing the function" even though he or she is able to do it. The Katz index is not scored, but it serves as a useful guide to client assessment.

Areas and Levels of Assessment

Bathing

Receives no assistance

Receives assistance bathing only one body part

Receives assistance bathing more than one part

Dressing

Gets clothing and dresses unassisted

Needs assistance tying shoes only

Needs assistance greater than above or stays undressed

Toileting

Requires no assistance

Needs assistance only in getting to toilet room or in cleaning self

Does not go to toilet room

Transferring

Needs no assistance from another person

Needs assistance transferring

Does not get out of bed

Continence

Continent

Occasional accident

Needs supervision, uses catheter, or is incontinent

Feeding

Needs no assistance

Needs assistance cutting meat and buttering bread

Needs more assistance or is tube or intravenously fed

Used with permission.

(The Gerontologist, Volume 10, No. 1, Spring 1970, Part 1, Page 23. © The Gerontological Society of America.)

The Lawton Instrumental Activities of Daily Living Scale

Instrumental activities of daily living (IADL's) are more complicated than self care tasks. Measurement of IADL's evaluates the client's ability to live independently in the community. The Lawton IADL scale is commonly used for geriatric client evaluation. A disadvantage to using this scale is that the scoring mechanism is unclear. However, use of the scale enables the nurse to identify clients who need help and determine which community resources will be useful to them.

A. Ability to use telephone   Score

1. Operates telephone on own initiative, looks up
   and dials numbers, etc.   1
2. Dials a few well-known numbers.   1
3. Answers telephone but does not dial.   1
4. Does not use telephone at all.   0

B. Shopping

1. Takes care of all shopping needs independently.   1
2. Shops independently for small purchases.   0
3. Needs to be accompanied on any shopping trip.   0
4. Completely unable to shop.   0

C. Food preparation

1. Plans, prepares, and serves adequate meals independently. — 1

2. Prepares adequate meals if supplied with ingredients. — 0

3. Heats, serves, and prepares meals or prepares meals but does not maintain adequate diet. — 0

4. Needs to have meals prepared and served. — 0

D. Housekeeping

1. Maintains house alone or with occasional assistance (e.g. heavy work, domestic help) — 1

2. Performs light daily tasks such as dishwashing, bed making. — 1

3. Performs light daily tasks but cannot maintain acceptable level of cleanliness. — 1

4. Needs help with all home maintenance tasks. — 1

5. Does not participate in any housekeeping tasks. — 1

E. Laundry

1. Does personal laundry completely. — 1

2. Launders small items, rinses stockings, etc. — 1

3. All laundry must be done by others. — 0

F. Mode of transportation

1. Travels independently on public transportation or drives own car. — 1

2. Arranges own travel via taxi but does not otherwise use public transportation. — 1

3. Travels on public transportation when accompanied by another.   1

4. Travel limited to taxi or automobile with assistance of another.   0

5. Does not travel at all.   0

G. Responsibility for taking own medications

1. Is responsible for taking medication in correct doses at correct time.   1

2. Takes responsibility if medication is prepared in advance in separate doses.   0

3. Is not capable of dispensing own medication.   0

H. Ability to handle finances

1. Manages financial matters independently (budgets, writes checks, pays rent and bills, goes to bank), collects and keeps track of income.   1

2. Manages day-to-day purchases but needs help with banking, major purchases, etc.   1

3. Incapable of handling money.   0

Score _____ (Out of possible 8)

(Modified from M.P. Lawton and E.M. Brody: "Assessment of Older People: Self-monitoring and Instrumental Activities of Daily Living," in Gerontologist, Vol. 9, pp. 179-186, 1969. Copyright by The Gerontological Society of America. Used with permission.)

(The Gerontologist, Volume 9, No. 3, 1969, Page 181. © The Gerontological Society of America)

THE HOLMES-RAHE SOCIAL ADJUSTMENT RATING SCALE

The Holmes-Rahe scale has become the guide for measuring stressors. Research produced using this scale shows a direct relationship between stress and illness.

Rank	Life Event	Life Change Units
1	Death of spouse	100
2	Divorce	73
3	Marital separation	65
4	Jail term	63
5	Death of close family member	63
6	Illness or personal injury	53
7	Marriage	50
8	Fired from job	47
9	Marital reconciliation	45
10	Retirement	45
11	Change in family member's health	44
12	Pregnancy	40
13	Sexual difficulties	39
14	Gain of new family member	39
15	Business readjustment	39
16	Change in financial state	38
17	Death of close friend	37
18	Change to different line of work	36
19	Change in number of arguments with spouse	35

20	Mortgage over $10,000	31
21	Foreclosure of mortgage or loan	30
22	Change in responsibilities at work	29
23	Son or daughter leaving home	29
24	Trouble with in-laws	29
25	Outstanding personal achievement	28
26	Spouse begins or stops work	26
27	Begin or end school	26
28	Change in living conditions	25
29	Revision of personal habits	24
30	Trouble with boss	23
31	Change in work hours or conditions	20
32	Change in residence	20
33	Change in school	20
34	Change in recreation	19
35	Change in church activities	19
36	Change in social activities	18
37	Mortgage or loan less than $10,000	17
38	Change in sleeping habits	16
39	Change in number of family get togethers	15
40	Change in eating habits	15
41	Vacation	13
42	Christmas	12
43	Minor violation of law	11

Scoring:

1-149	No significant life changes
150-199	Mild life changes with 33% chance of illness
200-299	Moderate life changes with 50% chance of illness
Over 300	Major life changes with 80% chance of illness.

HYPERTENSION

Hypertension is defined as sustained systolic blood pressure over 160 mm Hg. or diastolic blood pressure greater than 90 mm Hg. Diagnosis is based on blood pressure readings on at least two or more occasions.

Stages of Hypertension

Stage	Systolic blood pressure	Diastolic blood pressure
1	140-159	90-99
2	160-179	100-109
3	180-209	110-119
4	210 or higher	120 or higher

The blood pressure is measured with the client supine or sitting, then standing. The Joint National Committee study of 1992 recommends repeat blood pressure monitoring as follows:

- In one year, if systolic blood pressure is 130-139 and diastolic pressure is 85-89.

- In one month if client is in Stage 2.

- In one week if client is in Stage 3.

NORMAL JOINT RANGE OF MOTION

Assessment of joint range of motion is an important component of a restorative program. To determine the degree of impairment, the nurse must know the normal range of motion for each joint.

Neck

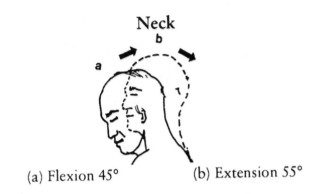

(a) Flexion 45°   (b) Extension 55°

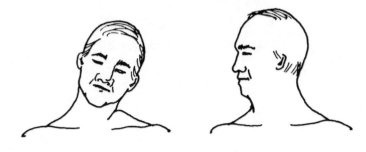

Lateral bending 40°   Rotation 70°

Elbow

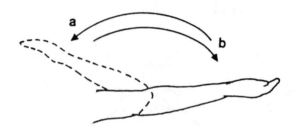

(a) Flexion 160°
(b) Extension 106° to 0°

Shoulder

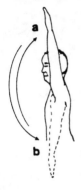

(a) Flexion 0° to160°
(b) Extension 160° to 0°

Knee

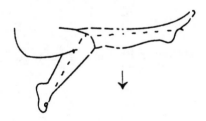

Flexion 120°

Fingers

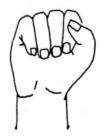

Flexion: Proximal phalange 90°
Middle phalange 120°
Distal phalange 80°

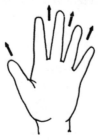

Extension: Proximal phalange 30°

Wrist

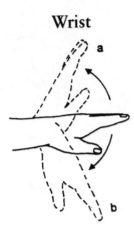

(a) Extension 70°   (b) Flexion 90°

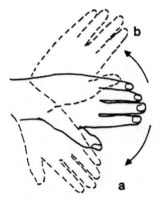

(a) Radial deviation 55°   (b) Ulnar deviation 20°

Hip

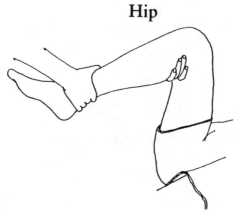

Flexion: (knee bent) 120°
(knee straight) 90°

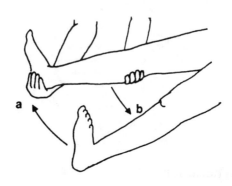

(a) Abduction 45°
(b) Adduction 40°

Ankle

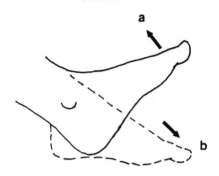

(a) Dorsi Flexion: 20°
(b) Plantar Flexion: 45°

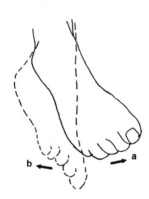

(a) Inversion: 30°   (b) Eversion 20°

Toes

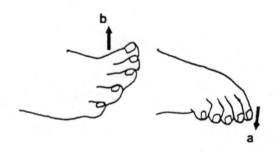

(a) Flexion: Distal phalange 50°
          Proximal phalange 35°

(b) Extension: Proximal phalange 80°

NURSING ASSESSMENT
RANGE OF MOTION FORM

Area	Right				Left			
Date								
Neck:								
Flexion (45°)								
Extension (55°)								
Lateral bending (40°)								
Rotation (70°)								
Shoulders:								
Flexion (160°)								
Extension (50°)								
Elbows:								
Flexion (160°)								
Extension (160° to 0°)								
Wrists:								
Flexion (90°)								
Extension (70°)								
Abduction (55°)								
Adduction (20°)								
Thumbs:								
Proximal phalange Flexion (70°)								
Distal phalange Flexion (90°)								

Continued…

Area	Right				Left			
Date								
Fingers:								
Proximal phalange Flexion (90°)								
Proximal phalange Extension (30°)								
Middle phalange Flexion (120°)								
Distal phalange Flexion (80°)								
Hips:								
Flexion (knee bent) (120°)								
Flexion (knee straight)(90°)								
Abduction (45°)								
Adduction (45°)								
Knees:								
Flexion (120°)								
Ankles:								
Dorsiflexion (20°)								
Plantar flexion (45°)								
Inversion (30°)								
Eversion (20°)								
Great Toe:								
Distal phalange Flexion (50°)								
Proximal phalange Flexion (35°)								
Extension (80°)								

HYDRATION

Intracellular fluid is lost with aging, resulting in a decrease in total body fluid. This reduces the margin of safety in fluid balance. Decreased fluid intake or increased fluid loss can quickly lead to fluid imbalance. Minimum fluid intake in the elderly should be no less than 1500ml to 1800ml per day. 2000ml to 3000ml daily is ideal. A general guideline for determining total daily baseline fluids is to multiply the client's body weight in kilograms times 30ml.

Signs and Symptoms of Dehydration

- Sunken cheeks
- Dry, brown tongue and mucous membranes
- Dry, inelastic skin
- Poor skin turgor
- Weight loss
- Hypotension
- Increased pulse
- Elevated temperature
- Weakness
- Mental confusion
- Concentrated urine
- BUN over 60 mg/dl
- Elevated serum creatinine
- Elevated hematocrit

Reasons for Inadequate Fluid Intake in the Elderly

Carefully evaluate the reason for decreased fluid intake in the elderly. Intake and output should balance within 200ml. Common reasons for inadequate fluid intake include:

- Fear of incontinence
- Age related changes in thirst sensation
- Lack of available fluid
- Physical or mental inability to consume fluids independently
- Depression, alteration in mood or cognitive status
- Gastrointestinal distress
- Apathy

Contributing Factors to Inadequate Hydration

- Nausea, vomiting, diarrhea
- Polyuria
- Increased metabolic rate/excessive activity
- Excessive perspiration
- Wound drainage
- Medication

Urine Specific Gravity

Measuring urine specific gravity is a simple, useful test to check for adequate hydration in the elderly. Using specific gravity testing for adequate hydration is particularly useful in the client's home, or long-term care setting. The urine specimen must be room temperature when it is tested. Normal adults with average fluid intakes will have urine specific gravity values that fluctuate between 1.016 and 1.022 during a 24 hour period. After 12 hours without fluid intake, urinary specific gravity is approximately 1.022. After 24 hours without fluids, specific gravity is 1.026. Urine becomes more concentrated and odor becomes stronger as specific gravity increases.

Elevated specific gravity values (1.022 or above, or according to agency policy) require further evaluation and intervention. Evaluate the client for clinical signs of dehydration. Follow agency policy for notifying attending physician, and performing glucose and protein dip stick tests. (Glucose and occasionally protein can occur in quantities sufficient to elevate the urine specific gravity.)

URINARY INCONTINENCE

Urinary incontinence is a major problem in the elderly. Incontinence is not a normal consequence of aging, and can frequently be cured or improved.

Causes of Urinary Incontinence

- Urinary tract infection
- Constipation or fecal impaction
- Medications, including diuretics
- Inadequate fluid intake
- Mental confusion
- Muscular weakness
- Environmental barriers
- Immobility related to acute or chronic disease
- Problems with clothing
- Estrogen depletion in females
- Prostate problems in males
- Chronic illness, disease, and trauma

Types of Urinary Incontinence

Type of Incontinence	Definition	Signs and Symptoms
Stress	Failure of urethral sphincter associated with increased intra-abdominal pressure	Urine loss during coughing, sneezing, laughing, postural changes, and physical activities
Urge	Involuntary loss of urine associated with a strong sense of urinary urgency.	Incontinence of urine with an abrupt and strong desire to void; involuntary sphinchter relaxation may cause involuntary loss of urine without symptoms.
Mixed incontinence	Combination of urge and stress incontinence.	Combination of urge and stress symptoms above; one symptom (urge or stress) may be more troublesome to client than the other.
Overflow	Overdistention of bladder.	Frequent or constant dribbling, urge or stress incontinence symptoms, urgency, frequency of urination.

Continued...

Type of Incontinence	Definition	Signs and Symptoms
Other functional	Chronic impairments of physical and/or cognitive functioning.	Urge incontinence or functional limitations.
Unconscious or reflux	Neurologic dysfunction.	Postvoiding or continuous incontinence; severe urgency with bladder hypersensitivity.

Client Management

1. Assessment of client
2. Assessment of type of incontinence
3. Treatment of reversible conditions
4. Discussion of incontinence treatment options
5. Implementation of plan of care consistent with client's condition, wishes, and goals
6. Education and quality of life improvement

Evaluation

1. History
   - Medical
   - Neurological
   - Genitourinary

- Review of risk factors
- Medications
- Review of symptoms of incontinence
- Duration and characteristics of incontinence
- Most troublesome symptom
- Frequency, timing, amount of continent voidings and incontinent episodes
- Precipitants of incontinence
- Other urinary tract symptoms (nocturia, dysuria, hesitancy, enuresis, straining, interrupted stream, pain)
- Bowel habits
- Daily fluid intake
- Alteration in sexual function due to incontinence
- Amount and type of protective devices used
- Previous treatments for incontinence and results
- Expectations of treatment

2. Mental status examination
    - Cognition
    - Motivation

3. Functional assessment
    - Dexterity
    - Mobility

4. Environmental assessment
5. Social Factors
   - Effect of incontinence on work
   - Effect of incontinence on relationships
   - Living arrangements
   - Identified caregiver and degree of caregiver's involvement
6. Bladder record
   - Frequency, timing, and amount of voiding
   - Amount of incontinent episodes
   - Activities associated with incontinence
   - Fluid intake
7. Physical examination
   - General examination
   - Abdominal examination
   - Rectal examination
   - Genital examination in male client
   - Pelvic examination in female client
   - Direct observation of urine loss with full bladder using stress test
   - Estimation of post void residual volume
   - Urinalysis
8. Supplemental assessments
   - Blood testing, chem profile

ASSESSMENT

Identification and Management of Reversible Causes of Incontinence

Potential Cause	Management
Urinary tract infection	Antibiotics
Atrophic urethritis/vaginitis	Estrogen replacement therapy
Postprostatectomy	Behavioral intervention. Avoid surgical intervention until it is evident that condition will not self-resolve.
Fecal impaction	Removal of impaction. Appropriate bowel regimen of stool softeners and bulk forming agents. Increase fiber in diet, increase fluid intake. Adequate exercise.
Metabolic hyperglycemia, hypercalcemia	Treat underlying condition. Implement retraining program.
Excess fluid intake	Treat underlying condition. Implement retraining program.
Volume overload	Treat underlying condition. Implement retraining program.
Venous insufficiency with edema	Treat underlying condition. Implement retraining program.
Congestive heart failure	Treat underlying condition. Implement retraining program.

Continued…

Potential Cause	Management
Psychological	Treat psychological disorder.
Impaired mobility	Treat underlying condition. Environmental assessment, facilitation of toileting facilities. Consider toileting aids and devices. Implement retraining program.

Drugs Affecting Urinary Incontinence

Urinary incontinence is the side effect of many drugs. Sometimes this is related to direct action of the drug, such as diuretics causing diuresis, which precipitates incontinence. Some drugs cause urinary retention, which may, over time, result in overflow incontinence. Other drugs may cause mental confusion in the elderly, causing secondary incontinence. A careful drug history of both prescription and over the counter drugs will assist with identification of these agents. In most cases, the drugs should be discontinued or changed, if clinically possible. Drugs that have the potential to cause incontinence include:

- Alcohol
- Anti-parkinson agents
- Anticholingergic agents
- Antidepressants

- Antihistamines
- Antispasmodics
- Beta-adrenergic agonists
- Caffeine
- Calcium channel blockers
- CNS depressants
- Disopyramide
- Diuretics
- Narcotic analgesics
- Phenothiazines
- Psychotropics
- Sedatives/hypnotics
- Sympathomimetics

Management Options

Target Population	Type of Intervention
Functionally disabled, Cognitively impared, Dependent, Incomplete bladder emptying	Scheduled toileting Habit training to match client's voiding habits
Caregiver dependent client, Recognizes urge to void, Physically able to use toilet, Able to request toileting assistance if required	Prompted voiding (scheduled voiding that requires prompting from caregiver)

Continued…

Target Population	Type of Intervention
Cognitively aware, recognizes urge to void, Able to learn how to inhibit urge, Physically able to toilet with or without assistance	Bladder training
Cognitively aware, Ability to identify and contract pelvic muscles, Complies with instructions	Pelvic muscle excercises
Ability to discern stimulation	Electrical stimulation useful as adjunct therapy in identification of pelvic muscles)
• Client ability to understand analog or digital signals using auditory or visual display • Motivated to learn through observation of biofeedback • Health care professional who can assess the incontinence problems and provide behavioral intervention	Biofeedback

Pharmacologic Options for Incontinence Management

Drug Classification	Indication
Anticholinergic agents	Urge incontinence
Alpha-adrenergic agents	Stress incontinence
Estrogen replacement	Stress or mixed incontinence

PRESSURE ULCERS

Definition: A pressure ulcer is any lesion caused by unrelieved pressure that results in damage to underlying tissue. Pressure ulcers usually occur over bony prominences and are graded or staged to classify the degree of tissue damage observed. Pressure ulcers do not necessarily progress from Stage I to Stage IV or heal from Stage IV to Stage I.

Stage I: Nonblanchable erythema of intact skin; the heralding lesion of skin ulceration. Note: Reactive hyperemia can normally be expected to be present for one half to three fourths as long as the pressure occluded the blood flow to the area; it should not be confused with a Stage I pressure ulcer.

Stage II: Partial thickness skin loss involving the epidermis and/or dermis. The ulcer is superficial and presents clinically as an abrasion, blister, or shallow crater.

Stage III: Full thickness skin loss involving damage or necrosis of subcutaneous tissue that may extend down to, but not through, underlying fascia. The ulcer presents clinically as a deep crater with or without undermining of adjacent tissue.

Stage IV: Full thickness skin loss with extensive destruction, tissue necrosis or damage to muscle, bone, or supporting structures (i.e., tendon or joint capsule). Note: Undermining and sinus tracts may also be associated with Stage IV pressure ulcers.

Prevention Measures

1. Systematically inspect skin daily, with particular attention to bony prominences; document findings.
2. Cleanse skin at time of soiling and at routine intervals; avoid hot water and use a mild cleansing agent.
3. Minimize environmental factors leading to drying; moisturize dry skin.

4. Avoid massage over bony prominences, which may increase tissue destruction.

5. Minimize skin exposure due to incontinence, perspiration, or wound drainage.

6. Avoid friction and shearing by using proper positioning, transferring, and turning techniques.

7. Provide an adequate intake of fluid, protein, and calories.

8. Improve the client's mobility status, if appropriate, and if indicated.

9. Reposition bedfast clients every two hours, or more often if indicted.

10. Use props and positioning devices to keep bony prominences from direct contact with one another.

11. Keep heels off the bed in bedfast clients.

12. Avoid positioning directly on the trochanter.

13. Use lifting devices to move clients in bed whenever possible.

14. Maintain the head of the bed at the lowest degree of elevation consistent with medical conditions and other restrictions.

15. Apply pressure reducing mattresses and pads to bed and chair.

16. Chair bound clients should be repositioned hourly. Clients who are able should be taught to shift their weight every 15 minutes.

17. Provide education to other health care providers, clients, and family or caregivers on the prevention of pressure ulcers.

Pressure Ulcer Management

1. Discuss treatment options with clients and their families.

2. Encourage clients to actively participate in their care.

3. Develop an effective plan of care consistent with client goals and wishes.

4. Implement a preventive program to prevent new areas from developing.

Pressure Ulcer Treatment Program

1. Assess the ulcer
   - Location
   - Stage
   - Size (length, width, depth)
   - Presence of sinus tracts, tunneling, undermining
   - Exudate
   - Presence or absence of necrosis
   - Presence or absence of granulation tissue and epithelialization

2. Evaluate the ulcer at the time of each treatment.; if the condition of the client or wound deteriorates, immediately reevaluate the treatment plan.

3. Reassess the ulcer weekly.

4. If no progress in healing is noted in 2 to 4 weeks, reevaluate the adequacy of the treatment plan, as well as adherence to this plan. Modify as needed.

5. Assess the client
   - Complete history and physical examination
   - Presence or absence of complicating conditions
   - Nutritional assessment
   - Pain assessment
   - Psychosocial assessment

6. Correct nutritional deficiencies

7. Provide pain management by eliminating mechanical sources of pain and providing analgesia.

8. Arrange interventions to meet identified psychosocial needs and goals.

9. Manage tissue loads
   - Positioning techniques and use of support surfaces

- Positioning devices
- Written schedules

Pressure Ulcer Care

1. Debride devitalized tissue by sharp, mechanical, enzymatic, or autolytic debridement.
2. Cleanse the wound
   - Avoid the use of skin cleansers and antiseptic agents that are cytotoxic.
   - Normal saline is an adequate skin cleanser for most pressure ulcers.
   - Use minimal mechanical force when cleansing the wound.
3. Apply a dressing appropriate to the wound type.
   - In general, the wound bed should be kept moist while surrounding tissue remains dry.
   - Control exudate but avoid desiccating the wound bed.
   - Loosely fill wound cavities with dressing material to avoid abscess formation.
   - Keep dressings intact

Management of Bacterial Colonization and Infection

1. Minimize colonization and enhance healing by effective cleansing and debridement.

2. Avoid swab cultures, which detect only surface colonization and may not reflect the true organism(s) causing tissue infection.

3. Consider topical antibiotic therapy trial in clean pressure ulcers that are not healing or are continuing to produce exudate after 2 to 4 weeks of treatment. If ineffective:

   • Consider osteomyelitis.

   • Perform quantitative tissue cultures by obtaining fluid through needle aspiration or tissue through ulcer biopsy.

4. Administer systemic antibiotics for clients with bacteremia, sepsis, advancing cellulitis, or osteomyelitis.

5. Avoid exogenous sources of contamination.

Infection Control

1. Apply the principles of standard precautions when treating pressure ulcers.

2. When treating multiple ulcers on the same client, treat the most contaminated ulcer last.

3. Use sterile instruments for debridement.

4. Follow agency policy for use of clean or sterile dressings; dispose of soiled dressings in a manner that avoids contamination.

Leg Ulcer Differentiation

Type of Ulcer	Cause of Ulcer	Signs and Symptoms
Venous	Venous hypertension (incompetent perforator valves)	• Irregular shape, surrounded by brown and blue pigmentation • Surrounding tissue often fibrotic • Wound usually flat or shallow crater • Varicosities • Edema • Exudate • Medial aspect of lower leg, typically just above medial malleolus of ankle • Pedal pulse usually present • Pain increases with leg dependency, decreases with cool environmental temperature, leg elevation, and activity
Arterial	Arteriosclerosis, atherosclerosis, peripheral vascular disease	• Lower leg, toes, heels, bony prominences of foot, rarely over medial malleolus of ankle • Well defined borders (continued...)

Type of Ulcer	Cause of Ulcer	Signs and Symptoms
Arterial (continued)		• Pale or white wound bed • Cool, atropic, shiny, hairless skin • Thick toenalis • Pedal pulse may be absent • Severe pain, decreases with leg dependency, increases with cool environment, activity, or leg elevation

Braden Scale

Bed and chair bound clients or those with impaired mobility should be assessed for factors that increase the risk of pressure sore development. Knowledge of the specific factors that place clients at risk is helpful. A systematic assessment can be accomplished by using a validated risk assessment tool, such as the Braden Scale. All risk assessments should be documented. Pressure ulcer risk assessment should be repeated periodically.

The Braden Scale scoring is as follows:

High Risk: Total score ≤12

Moderate Risk: Total score 13-14

Low Risk: Total score 15-16 if under 75 years old or 15-18 if over 75 years old

BRADEN SCALE — For Predicting Pressure Sore Risk

Risk Factor	Score / Description				Date of Assess.			
					1	2	3	4
SENSORY PERCEPTION Ability to respond meaningfully to pressure-related discomfort	1. COMPLETELY LIMITED– Unresponsive (does not moan, flinch, or grasp) to painful stimuli, due to diminished level of consciousness or sedation, OR limited ability to feel pain over most of body surface.	2. VERY LIMITED– Responds only to painful stimuli. Cannot communicate discomfort except by moaning or restlessness, OR has a sensory impairment which limits the ability to feel pain or discomfort over 1/2 of the body.	3. SLIGHTLY LIMITED– Responds to verbal commands but cannot always communicate discomfort or need to be turned OR has some sensory impairment which limits ability to feel pain or discomfort in 1 or 2 extremities.	4. NO IMPAIRMENT– Responds to verbal commands. Has no sensory deficit which would limit ability to feel or voice pain or discomfort.				
MOISTURE Degree to which skin is exposed to moisture	1. CONSTANTLY MOIST– Skin is kept moist almost constantly by perspiration, urine, etc. Dampness is detected every time patient is moved or turned.	2. OFTEN MOIST – Skin is often moist but not always moist. Linen must be changed at least once a shift.	3. OCCASIONALLY MOIST– Skin is occasionally moist, requiring an extra linen change approximately once a day.	4. RARELY MOIST– Skin is usually dry; linen only requires changing at routine intervals.				
ACTIVITY Degree of physical activity	1. BEDFAST– Confined to bed.	2. CHAIRFAST– Ability to walk severely limited or nonexistant. Cannot bear own weight and/or must be assisted into chair or wheelchair.	3.WALKS OCCA-SIONALLY– Walks occasionally during day but for very short distances, with or without assistance. Spends majority of each shift in bed or chair.	4. WALKS FREQUENTLY– Walks outside the room at least twice a day and inside room at least once every 2 hours during waking hours.				

BRADEN SCALE — For Predicting Pressure Sore Risk (part 2)

Risk Factor	Score / Description				Date of Assess.			
					1	2	3	4
MOBILITY Ability to change and control body position	1. COMPLETELY IMMOBILE– Does not make even slight changes in body or extremity position without assistance.	2. VERY LIMITED– Makes occasional slight changes in body or extremity position but unable to make frequent or significant changes independently.	3. SLIGHTLY LIMITED– Makes frequent though slight changes in body or extremity position independently.	4. NO LIMITATIONS– Makes major and frequent changes in position without assistance.				
NUTRITION Usual food intake pattern	1. VERY POOR– Never eats a complete meal. Rarely eats more than 1/3 of any food offered. Eats 2 servings or less of protein (meat or dairy products) per day. Takes fluids poorly. Does not take a liquid dietary supplement OR is NPO1 and/or maintained on clear liquids or IV2 for more than 5 days.	2. PROBABLY INADEQUATE – Rarely eats a complete meal and generally eats only about 1/2 of any food offered. Protein intake includes only 3 servings of meat or dairy products per day. Occasionally will take a dietary supplement, OR receives less than optimum amount of liquid diet or tube feeding.	3. ADEQUATE– Eats over 1/2 of most meals. Eats a total of 4 servings of protein (meat, dairy products) each day. Occasionally will refuse a meal, but will usually take a supplement if offered, OR is on tube feeding or TPN3 regimen, which probably meets most of nutritional needs.	4. EXCELLENT– Eats most of every meal. Never refuses a meal. Usually eats a total of 4 or more servings of meat and dairy products. Occasionally eats between meals. Does not require supplementation.				
1NPO: Nothing by mouth 2IV: Intravenously 3TPN: Total parenteral nutrition.								

CONTINUED...

BRADEN SCALE — For Predicting Pressure Sore Risk (part 3)

Risk Factor	Score / Description			Date of Assess.				
					1	2	3	4
FRICTION AND SHEAR	1. PROBLEM– Requires moderate to maximum assistance in moving. Complete lifting without sliding against sheets is impossible. Frequently slides down in bed or chair, requiring frequent repositioning with maximum assistance. Spasticity, contractures, or agitation leads to almost constant friction.	2. POTENTIAL PROBLEM– Moves feebly or requires minimum assistance. During a move, skin probably slides to some extent against sheets, chair, restraints, or other devices. Maintains relatively good position in chair or bed most of the time but occasionally slides down.	3. NO APPARENT PROBLEM– Moves in bed and in chair independently and has sufficient muscle strength to lift up completely during move. Maintains good position in bed or chair at all times.					
Total Score	Total Score of 12 or less represents HIGH RISK							

NEUROLOGICAL CHECKS

Neurological checks are performed in many different conditions where neurological disorder or injury is suspected. Neuro checks are normally documented on a flow sheet. The following points are essential to a thorough assessment.

Level of consciousness

Level of consciousness is the most important indicator of cerebral injury.

Alert	(Client awake and responds appropriately)
Lethargic	(Very sleepy, but arouses to stimulation)
Obtunded	(Difficult to arouse, but responds appropriately)
Stuporous	(Not completely alert, responds to pain)
Semicomatose	(Reflex movements, responds to pain)
Comatose	(No response)

Orientation

Person
Place
Time
Situation

Judgment

Coherent

Thoughts distorted

Appropriate verbal response

Memory

Short term

Past

long-term

Affect

Alert

Pleasant

Restricted

Dull

Speech

Aphasia

Dysphasia

Articulate

Appropriate

Pain

Reaction to stimulation

Reaction to painful stimulation

Pupil Assessment

Equal

Reactive/Nonreactive

Sluggish

Motor

Decerebrate

Decorticate

GLASGOW COMA SCALE

The Glasgow coma scale is used for monitoring neurologic dysfunction. The test is scored by adding the total of all three categories. The examiner determines the best response the client can make to stimuli. Higher point values are assigned to responses that indicate increasing degrees of awareness and arousal. A total score of less than 8 indicates a neurological crisis. A total of 9-13 indicates moderate dysfunction, and a score of 13-15 indicates moderate to minor dysfunction.

Eyes Open

Spontaneously	4
To Speech	3
To Pain	2
No Response	1

Verbal Response

Oriented and Talking	5
Disoriented/Talking	4
Words Unintelligible	3
Moaning/Groaning	2
No Verbalization	1

Motor Response

Obeys commands	6
Localizes pain	5
Flexion: Withdrawal	4
Decorticate:Flexion	3
Decerebrate: Rigidity	2
No Response	1

(Hickey, J: The Clinical Practice of Neurological Nursing, JB Lippincott, 1981. Used with permission by Lippincott-Raven Publishers.)

INCIDENCE AND PREVALENCE OF SEIZURES IN THE ELDERLY

Seizures, epilepsy, and status epilepticus occur with increasing frequency in the elderly. Idiopathic seizures are those with no identifiable cause. Symptomatic seizures have an identifiable cause. Although idiopathic seizures can occur in the elderly, most seizures occur as the result of an identifiable cause. Common causes of seizures in the elderly include:

- Epilepsy
- Electrolyte imbalance
- Cerebral infarction
- Cerebral anoxia
- Head trauma
- Intracranial infection
- Alcohol or drug withdrawal
- Reduction or withdrawal of anticonvulsant drugs
- Drug toxicity
- Hypoglycemia
- Hypocalcemia
- Hyponatremia
- Uremia
- Brain tumor
- Subdural hematoma
- Cortical vein thrombosis
- Third degree heart block or other cardiac dysrhythmia

SEIZURE CHARACTERISTICS

Type of Seizure	Signs of Seizure Activity	Comment
Generalized Tonic-Clonic (Grand Mal Seizure)	May be preceded by an aura. Loss of conciousness, convulsive activity, characterized by rigid stiffening of muscles and jerking movement of the arms and legs. Excessive salivation. Cyanosis due to lack of oxygen, incontinence of bowel and bladder.	Usually lasts 3 to 4 minutes. Post-ictally, the client may be very tired and have a headache, mental confusion, slurred speech, weakness. The client will not remember the seizure.
Absence Seizure (Petit Mal Seizure)	Staring, blinking, or stopping what the client is doing. May stare blankly. One muscle group may twitch or jerk.	Usually last less than a minute, but may occur many times a day.
Simple-Partial (Jacksonian)	Muscle spasms of the face, hands, or feet. Starts in one extremity, such as an arm or leg, and progressively moves upward on that side of the body.	May spread to other areas in the brain, resulting in a generalized tonic-clonic seizure.

Continued...

Type of Seizure	Signs of Seizure Activity	Comment
Complex-Partial (Psychomotor)	Abnormal acts, irrational behavior or loss of judgment due to a temporary change in consciousness. Automatic behavior may continue normally. May uncontrollably twitch part of body.	Usually lasts only a few seconds. The client usually does not remember the seizure.
Myoclonic	Consists of one or more myoclonic jerks. The client remains conscious but cannot control the muscle movement.	The client is aware that an extremity is jerking but is unable to stop it. Remains conscious throughout and can remember the seizure activity.
Status Epilepticus	Multiple seizures occurring simultaneously with no break between seizures.	Status epilepticus may be precipitated by sudden withdrawal of anti-seizure medications, fever, and infection. This type of seizure is dangerous and can lead to decreased mental function, neurological impairment, and death.

HYPOTHERMIA

The elderly are predisposed to hypothermia due to aging changes that impair the body's thermoregulatory responses. Clients with diseases such as diabetes, Parkinson's disease, or cerebrovascular diseases appear to be at higher risk. Hypothermia may be drug induced by alcohol, barbiturates, phenothiazines, tricyclic antidepressants, benzodiazepines, anesthetics, and narcotics. The elderly can become hypothermic in warm climates.

Socioeconomic and environmental conditions may also predispose the elderly to accidental hypothermia. Many elderly adults are socially isolated. Some lack a central heating system. Many are on limited budgets and may not heat their residence adequately.

Hypothermia may be mistaken for drug or alcohol abuse, hypoglycemia, a post-ictal state, new stroke, or hypothyroidism. Some clients may not be able to tell you they are cold. Others with impaired thermoregulatory ability will not realize they are cold. Signs and symptoms of the various stages of hypothermia may be vague in the elderly. If a client presents with any of the listed symptoms, hypothermia should be ruled out.

ASSESSMENT

Mild hypothermia

- Core body temperature 90°-95°F(32°-35°C)
- Apathy
- Weakness
- Fatigue
- Slurred speech
- Mental confusion
- Slowed gait
- Skin cool to touch
- Facial edema
- Pale or ashen skin
- Tachypnea

Moderate Hypothermia

- Core body temperature 82°-90°F (28°-32°C)
- Mental confusion progresses to loss of consciousness as temperature drops
- Slow reflexes
- Sluggish pupils
- Muscle stiffness
- Involuntary tremor
- Skin cold to touch
- Cyanosis
- Pulse, respiration, blood pressure decrease

- As temperature drops, spontaneous dysrhythmias occur; most common are sinus bradycardia and atrial fibrillation.

Severe Hypothermia

- Core temperature below 82°F (28°C)
- Client may appear to be dead
- Skin cold to touch
- Unresponsiveness
- Pupils fixed and dilated
- Muscles rigid, areflexic
- Respirations cease
- Oliguria
- Anuria

ALTERED PRESENTATION OF SPECIFIC ILLNESSES IN THE OLDER ADULT

The elderly client's body may not respond to illness in the same manner as that of the younger adult. Signs and symptoms of disease may not be as well defined. Occasionally the presenting symptoms appear unrelated to the underlying problem. Expected signs and symptoms may not be present at all. Atypical presentations of common disorders in the elderly are listed as follows.

Problem/Condition	Possible Signs & Symptoms in the Elderly
Depression	All classic symptoms of depression, plus concentration and memory disturbances, increased somnolence, weight gain.
Urinary tract infection	Frequency, urgency, nocturia may be present. Dysuria frequently absent. Incontinence, mental confusion, and anorexia are additional signs.
Myocardial Infarction	No chest pain or atypical pain in jaw, neck, shoulder. Shortness of breath, tachypnea, hypotension, arrhythmia, restlessness, syncope.
Congestive heart failure	Restlessness, confusion, anorexia, cyanosis.

INITIATING AN ASSESSMENT FOR DEMENTIA

A diagnosis of dementia requires evidence of decline from previous levels of functioning and impairment in multiple cognitive domains (see Diagnostic and Statistical Manual of Mental Disorders, Fourth Edition [DSM-IV], American Psychiatric Association, 1994).

An initial assessment is necessary to determine whether a client's symptoms meet the current criteria for dementia. The initial assessment should combine information from several sources. The components of the assessment should include:

- Focused history
- Physical examination
- Mental status assessment

Focused History

The history should document the chronology of the problem and include:

- Chief complaint
- Mode of onset (rapid versus gradual)
- Progression
- Duration of symptoms

ASSESSMENT

Medical History

- Relevant systemic diseases
- Psychiatric disorders
- Known neurological disorders
- History of head injury
- Alcohol or substance abuse
- Exposure to environmental toxins
- Intercurrent, infectious, or metabolic illness

Family History

- History of Alzheimer's disease
- History of other conditions which lead to dementia (e.g. Parkinson's Disease)

Social and Cultural History

- Recent life events
- Social support network
- Education
- Literacy
- Socioeconomic background
- Ethnic background
- Cultural background

Medication History

- Prescription drugs
- Over the counter drug use
- Alcohol
- Herbs, vitamins, and other natural substances

Informant Reports

- Interview the client alone first
- Inform the client that others will be interviewed
- Interview informants separately from client
- Consider the possibility of questionable motives to informant's reports.

Focused Physical Examination

- Use standard principles to conduct a focused physical examination
- Carefully assess for conditions that cause delirium
- Be alert to signs of abuse and neglect

Functional Status Assessment

The Functional Activities Questionnaire is an informant-based measure of the client's abilities.

Levels of performance on the Functional Activities Questionnaire are assigned as follows:

- Dependent=3
- Requires assistance=2
- Has difficulty but does by self=1
- Normal=0
- Never did the activity, but could do it=0
- Never did the activity and would have difficulty doing it now=1

Maximum Score   **Score**

Orientation

Maximum Score	Score	
3	( )	Can the client write checks, pay bills, balance the check book?
3	( )	Can the client assemble tax records, business affairs, or papers?
3	( )	Can the client shop alone for clothing, household items, or groceries?
3	( )	Can the client play a game of skill or work on a hobby?
3	( )	Can the client heat water, make a cup of coffee, and turn on the stove?

3	( )	Can the client prepare a balanced meal?
3	( )	Can the client keep track of current events?
3	( )	Can the client pay attention to, understand and discuss TV, books, and magazines?
3	( )	Can the client travel out of the neighborhood, drive, or arrange to take the bus?

Score _____

A total score for the questionnaire is computed by adding the scores across the ten items. Scores range from 0 to 30. A cutpoint of "9" (dependent in three or more activities) is recommended.

Mental Status Evaluation

The client's medical history will provide clues to current mental status, but a separate tool is needed to determine and document it. Preface the examination by asking the client's permission to ask questions about how he/she feels and thinks. Be empathetic in conducting the cognitive examination to avoid emotional responses to failures.

Name

Age

Appearance

- Self neglect
- Ability/inability to dress
- Level of activity/body mannerisms
- Gait
- Sensory aids, such as glasses or hearing aid
- Signs of lethargy

Speech

- Rapid
- Slow
- Clear
- Slurred
- Aphasia
- Difficulty naming objects

Mood, feelings, behavior, and attitude

- Cooperative
- Cheerful
- Optimistic
- Overconfident

- Hopelessness
- Depression
- Worthlessness
- Guilt
- Mood associated disturbances of appetite or sleep
- Overwhelming dread or sense of impending doom
- Apathy
- Irritability
- Hostility
- Indifference
- Suspicion

Obsessions or compulsions

- Recurrent unwanted ideas
- Recurrent unwanted behavior

Hallucinations

- Visual
- Auditory
- Gustatory
- Somatic complaints

Phobias

- Irrational fears

Cognition

- Attention
- Orientation
- Memory, recent and remote
- Concrete thought processes
- Abstract thought processes
- Language function

Content of thought

- Replies spontaneous
- Preoccupied
- Ideas of reference
- Looseness of association
- Delusions

Judgment

Decision making ability

- Problem solving
- Intellectual functioning/knowledge

Coping ability

- Use of defense mechanisms
- Accepts responsibility for own actions
- Stress-crisis cycle

Mini-Mental Status Evaluation

A mental status evaluation should be conducted on every client. This tool, developed by Folstein, is simple and practical and can be completed in a short amount of time. The tool may be used as part of the admission assessment. It can also be done daily or weekly to track a client's deterioration or recovery. It is useful in cerebrovascular accidents, AIDS-related lymphomas, and other neurological disorders. A score greater than 24 is considered normal. Scores below 24 are associated with delirium, dementia, or severe depression.

Maximum Score	Score	
		Orientation
5	( )	What is the date? (year, season, day, month)
5	( )	Where are we? (city, state, hospital, floor)

ASSESSMENT

Registration

3   ( )   Name 3 objects.
Speak slowly allowing one
second for each object.
Repeat the list until all three
are learned. One point for
each correct answer.
Count and record trials.

Number of trials _____

Attention and Calculation

5   ( )   Serial 7's. One point for
each correct. Stop after 5
answers. Alternatively, spell
"world" backwards.

Recall

3   ( )   Ask for the 3 objects repeated
above. One point for
each correct answer.

Language

9   ( )   Name a pencil, and watch.
Repeat the following: "No
ifs and's or but's." (1 point)

Follow a 3 stage command:

"Take a paper in your right hand, fold it in half, and put it on the floor." (3 points)

Have the client read and obey the following:

1	( )	Close your eyes. (1 point)
1	( )	Write a sentence. (1 point)
1	( )	Copy design. (1 point)
	( )	Total score

Assess level of consciousness along a continuum:

<u>Alert</u>   <u>Drowsy</u>   <u>Stupor</u>   <u>Coma</u>

Used with permission.

(Folstein, MF and SE: Journal of Psychiatric Research, Volume 12, pages 189–198, Elsevier Science, Ltd., Pergamon Imprints134

, Oxford, England, 1975.)

CAUSES OF ACUTE CONFUSIONAL STATES IN THE ELDERLY

Mental confusion is not a normal consequence of aging, and is often caused by reversible conditions. Carefully assess confused clients for the following conditions:

- Vascular insufficiency
- Central nervous system infection
- Trauma

- Tumors
- Cardiovascular disease, including decreased cardiac output, alteration in peripheral vascular resistance, congestive heart failure, and vascular occlusion
- Hypotension
- Pulmonary disorders, including inadequate gas exchange and infection
- Systemic infections, acute and chronic
- Metabolic disorders, including electrolyte imbalance, acidosis/alkalosis, hyper and hypoglycemia, and volume depletion
- Anemias
- Decreased renal function
- Drug toxicity
- Endocrine system disorders
- Nutritional deficiencies, malnutrition
- Emotional stress
- Pain
- Surgery, anesthesia
- Alteration in temperature regulation
- Dehydration
- Depression
- Anxiety

- Grief
- Fatigue
- Sensory/perceptual deficits
- Unfamiliar environment
- Sensory deprivation
- Sensory overload
- Immobility
- Exposure to toxic substances

DEPRESSION

Depression in older adults is frequently overlooked and untreated. Depression is the most common functional mental illness seen in the elderly. Symptoms of depression in the elderly can include cognitive changes that may be mistaken for delirium or dementia. A thorough assessment is necessary to determine the cause of the symptoms.

Geriatric Depression Scale (Short Form)

Directions: Answer yes or no to each of the following questions. Choose the answer that best describes the way you have felt over the past week.

	Yes	No
1. Are you basically satisfied with your life?	____	____
2. Have you dropped many of your activities and interests?	____	____
3. Do you feel that your life is empty?	____	____
4. Do you often get bored?	____	____
5. Are you in good spirits most of the time?	____	____
6. Are you afraid that something bad is going to happen to you?	____	____
7. Do you feel happy most of the time?	____	____
8. Do you often feel helpless?	____	____
9. Do you prefer to stay at home, rather than going out and doing new things?	____	____

10. Do you feel that you have more
    problems with memory
    than most?   ____   ____

11. Do you think it is wonderful
    to be alive now?   ____   ____

12. Do you feel pretty worthless
    the way you are now?   ____   ____

13. Do you feel full of energy?   ____   ____

14. Do you feel that your
    situation is hopeless?   ____   ____

15. Do you think that most people
    are better off than you are?   ____   ____

Interpretation: Score_____

Scoring: Add up all the yes answers. A higher score
indicates more depressive symptoms. A score of 5 or
greater suggests depression and should be evaluated.

DEPRESSION IN THE ELDERLY

Depression in the elderly frequently occurs as a result of failing physical health and numerous losses. It is often difficult to differentiate from other conditions and may be unrecognized. Both health care workers and clients may attribute symptoms of depression to the aging process. In the elderly, these symptoms may present as somatic complaints and are easily overlooked. Instead of complaining of depressed mood, the elderly often complain of anorexia, sleep disturbance, lack of energy, and loss of interest and enjoyment in life.

Symptoms of dementia may mask depression. The reverse is also true. The depressed client may present with symptoms that appear to be dementia, such as disorientation, distractability, and memory loss. Careful assessment and differential diagnosis are essential.

The current American Psychiatric Association Diagnostic and Statistical Manual (DSM-IIIR) criteria for depression include:

- weight and appetite changes
- sleep disturbances
- motor agitation or retardation
- lack of energy and fatigue
- irritable or depressed mood
- lack of interest in usual activities
- feelings of worthlessness, excessive guilt, or self-reproach

- suicidal ideation or attempts
- difficulty concentrating or thinking

To establish the diagnosis of major depression, the DSM-IIIR requires the presence for at least five of the symptoms listed.

A 1988 study on suicide in the elderly showed that the suicide rate was higher than that for the general population. This study showed the suicide rate for the general population as 12.4/100,000, compared with rates in 80 to 84 year olds as 26.5/100,000[1]. Elderly males were deemed the highest risk for completed suicides. In the study group, more than three fourths had visited their primary health care provider within 30 days of their suicide.

The incidence of major depression in nursing home residents is also high and frequently unrecognized. According to the Epidemiologic Catchment Area Study, depressive symptoms occur in 15 to 25 percent of residents in nursing homes. The rates of newly diagnosed major depression in long term care were identified as occurring in 13 percent of residents over a one year period. Another 18 percent were identified as having new depressive symptoms[2]. The OBRA long term care regulations require facilities to ensure that residents who display mental or psychosocial adjustment difficulties receive appropriate treatment and services. However, long term care facilities may not screen for depression, or have staff capability for appropriate or timely interventions. This problem may be compounded by misinterpretation of other OBRA regulations regarding the use (and avoidance) of drugs deemed to be chemical restraints.

Consequences of Unrecognized/Untreated Depression in the Elderly Include:

- Despair, suffering, feelings of isolation, lost status, and loss of personal happiness
- Family members and significant others failure to understand the condition and provide support for the client
- Professional help is not sought in a timely manner, if at all
- Untreated depression is likely to persist indefinitely
- Severe strain on living circumstances, which may cause a shift from living at home to a nursing facility
- Higher health care costs because unrecognized depression creates the need for more medical services related to physical illnesses

Steps in Detecting and Treating Depressive Conditions

- Evaluate risk factors
- Maintain a high index of awareness of how insidious geriatric depression can be and screen accordingly
- Utilize a self report questionnaire and evaluate in con-

junction with information about depressive symptoms obtained in the clinical interview

- Identify mood syndrome by clinical history, interview, report by spouse or significant other
- Identify potential known causes of mood syndrome, such as medical, medications, alcohol or substance abuse, and other causal non-mood psychiatric disorders
- Conduct appropriate client/family teaching related to the condition, medications, and treatment
- Refer to an appropriate health care professional
- Assist in the treatment of potential causes
- Reevaluate for mood symptoms/mood persistence

In assessing the client for depression, confounding problems, use of selected prescription medications, and alcohol or substance abuse must also be considered. Confounding factors in diagnosis and treatment of depression in the geriatric client include:

- Concurrent psychotropic medications, which may:
  - Cause the client to become depressed
  - Change blood levels of antidepressants
  - Increase side effects of antidepressants
  - Biochemically block the effects of antidepressant medications
  - Require modification of the oral dosage
- Concurrent medical problems, which may:
  - Cause depression biologically

- Decrease the efficacy of psychotherapy and antidepressant medication
- Change drug metabolism of antidepressants
- Impair the client's ability to participate in treatment
- Contribute to both chronicity of depression and reduced efficacy of treatment
- Increase the need for simplified dosing schedules for medication self administration (e.g. once daily)
- Concurrent non-mood psychiatric conditions, which may:
  - Cause depression, as in early Alzheimer's disease
  - Require different medications
  - Reduce client's ability to participate in treatment
  - Reduce the response to antidepressants
  - Worsen the prognosis of depression (e.g. alcoholism or substance abuse)
- Other issues:
  - The client's metabolism slows during the aging process, which may create the need for lower drug dosages
  - Transportation problems may restrict the client's access to care
  - The client may require more time for interview and/or assessment
  - The client's fixed income, high co-pays, or reim-

bursement constraints may limit the client's access
to assistance and necessitate a referral
- Fixed income may limit availability of therapy and
nongeneric medications

Obstacles to treatment of depression in the geriatric client include:

- Stigma present amongst the elderly regarding mental illness and psychiatric treatment
- The client may not report the condition unless directly questioned because he/she mistakes the symptoms as part of the aging process, or because of no hope of help
- Unwillingness of health care workers to listen to the client's concerns
- Lack of understanding of health care providers regarding the cause and nature of geriatric depression
- Clients do not present their complaint to their primary health care provider in a manner that make the diagnosis and treatment of depression apparent
- Lack of understanding/client teaching about depression and it's course by clients and families
- Lack of understanding/client teaching about the importance of taking medications as ordered
- Lack of compliance with medication regimen
- Concurrent medical illnesses interfering with antidepressant response

- Alcohol or substance abuse
- Life stressors causing client noncompliance with treatment regimen
- Lack of access to services related to financial constraints, inadequate Medicare reimbursement to physicians, or restrictions on treatment by HMO's, PPO's, and private health insurance plans

Goals of treatment for depression include:

- Partial or complete improvement in symptoms
- Reduced risk of recurrance and relapse
- Improved quality of life
- Improved medical health, and relief of pain and suffering associated with physical illnesses
- Enhancement of mental and physical well-being and social functioning
- Minimization of cognitive disability
- Decreased mortality

(The Beck Depression Inventory is an excellent tool for assessing depression. It does not appear in this text due to the copyright holder's guidelines prohibiting reproduction of the tool in it's entirety. For information on obtaining the Beck Depression Inventory, please contact the Psychological Corporation at 1-800-211-8378.)

---

[1]Diagnosis and Treatment of Depression in Late Life, National Institutes of Health Consensus Development Conference Statement, November 4-6, 1991

[2]Diagnosis and Treatment of Depression in Late Life, National Institutes of Health Consensus Development Conference Statement, November 4-6, 1991

DIFFERENTIATION OF DELIRIUM, DEPRESSION, AND DEMENTIA

Delirium: An acute confusional state caused by a variety of treatable illnesses or conditions. Delirium may be caused by an adverse reaction to medication. Delirium is a serious problem which may be unrecognized or mistaken for the natural progression of dementia. If unrecognized and untreated, the morbidity and mortality is high.

Depression: A mental state characterized by depressed mood, sadness, discouragement, and despair. Depression is frequently diagnosed, particularly when the client is physically ill. Diagnosis may be complicated because depression may be mistaken for dementia (and vice-versa), each may present as the other, and they may coexist. Alteration in memory, attention, and executive function suggest depression. Marked visuospatial or language impairment suggests dementia.. Drug interactions (polypharmacy) can produce depression and contribute to cognitive impairment.

Dementia: An organic mental disorder characterized by loss of intellectual capabilities involving impairment of memory, judgment, abstract thinking, and personality changes.

	Delirium	Depression	Dementia
Onset	Sudden	Gradual or rapid	Gradual
Orientation	Fluctuating level of awareness, disorientation, clouding of sensorium, decline in level of consciousness	Oriented or disoriented	Disoriented
Behavior	Agitation or apathy, inability to perform ADL's	Apathy, agitation, change in appetite, self neglect	Agitation, inability to perform ADL's, changes in sleep-wake cycle

Continued…

	Delirium	Depression	Dementia
Onset	Sudden	Gradual or rapid	Gradual
Affect	Varies	Despair, worry	Labile, flat
Speech	May be incoherent and inappropriate or coherent and appropriate	Coherent, may not want to talk	Repetitive; initially may lie to cover problem. In later stage does not conceal deficits
Prognosis	Good; resolves with treatment	Good; resolves with treatment of cause or with treatment of depression	Poor; unable to reverse cause

MAJOR FORMS OF DEMENTIA

Disease	Description	Course of Illness
Alzheimer's	Diagnosis by exclusion of other disorders; neuritic plaques and neurofibrillary tangles noted on autopsy. Strong familial tendency.	Onset age 55-70; outcome variable depending on damage to brain cells.
Huntington's Disease	Hereditary; degeneration of the cerebral cortex and basal ganglia	Onset age 25-45; slowly progressive.
Pick's Disease	Atrophy of frontal and temporal lobes	Onset age 40-60, progressive. Similar to Alzheimer's Disease
Creutzfeldt-Jacob Disease	Noninflammatory virus	Onset age 50-60; rapidly progressive-usually 6-12 months.
AIDS Dementia	HIV infection of central nervous system	May be the first sign of illness in 10% of AIDS patients; early symptoms often difficult to distinguish from depression.

SLEEP PROBLEMS IN THE ELDERLY

The elderly frequently complain of difficulty sleeping and daytime drowsiness. Many elderly clients take prescription sleeping medications.

Characteristics of Sleep in the Elderly

1. The older adult awakens briefly numerous times during the night.
2. There is a loss of deepest levels of stage 3 and 4 deep sleep (non-REM sleep) in the elderly.
3. The elderly nap more during the day than other age groups.
4. Body temperature normally drops during sleep. The elderly have less of a drop in body temperature than younger adults.
5. Most elderly clients prefer earlier bedtimes. Likewise, they prefer earlier wake-up.

Causes of Sleep Disorders in the Elderly

1. Sleep apnea is more common in the elderly. It is more prevalent in men than in women.
2. The elderly have a increased incidence of myoclonic activity (muscle jerking) during sleep. The myoclonic activity briefly wakens the client.

3. Medical problems such as heart failure, breathing problems, gastric reflux and chronic pain prevent many clients from sleeping well.

4. Psychiatric disorders and dementia commonly impair sleep.

5. Sundowning increases agitation and disorientation in the evening and night. It occurs frequently in dementia and is a major reason for nursing home placement due to family inability to deal with the behavior.

6. Poor sleep habits, such as erratic sleep schedules, nicotine, caffeine, alcohol ingestion, spending too much time in bed, and uncomfortable sleeping environment frequently lead to impaired sleep.

7. A common cause of impaired sleep is the inappropriate use of sleeping pills. Many drugs have the opposite of the intended effect in the elderly.

8. The elderly frequently complain of sleep problems because they do not sleep as well as they did when they were younger.

Assessment of Sleep Problems in the Elderly

1. Ask the client to keep a 24 hour journal of sleep/wake times for 5 days.

2. Ask a family member or caregiver to observe

the client's breathing during sleep for signs of sleep apnea, which is manifested by snoring and periods of apnea.

3. Assess for cardiac dysrhythmias.

4. Assess body temperature abnormalities.

Treatment of Sleep Problems in the Elderly

1. Provide a comfortable sleeping environment. Avoid temperature extremes.

2. Advise the client to avoid nicotine, alcohol, caffeine. Limit liquids in the evening.

3. Advise the client to use the bedroom for sleep only. Use other areas of the house for watching television and reading.

4. Treat underlying medical problems which are interfering with sleep.

5. Manage psychiatric problems which are interfering with sleep.

6. Avoid routine use of sleeping pills.

7. Educate the client that less effective sleep is common in the elderly. Teach that the elderly have different sleeping patterns than younger adults.

8. Adhere to a regular bedtime and arousal time.

9. Avoid daytime naps.

10. The sleep laboratory can perform a comprehensive evaluation in which the client's sleep is monitored for one or more nights. A sleep lab evaluation should be performed if:

   a. The client snores heavily and has daytime sleepiness. (Suggests sleep apnea).

   b. The client or spouse notices restless legs during sleep. (Evidence of myoclonic activity).

   c. There is a disturbance in sleep phase cycle.

   d. Other avenues of treatment are not effective.

FALL RISK CONSIDERATIONS

- History of falls during previous year
- Recent surgery
- Dizziness/other balance problem
- Unsteady gait
- Joint immobility related to arthritis or injury
- Fatigue
- Weakness
- Paresis/paralysis
- Seizure disorder
- Vision impairment

- Hearing impairment
- Mental confusion
- Impaired judgment
- Inability to understand/follow directions
- Unfamiliar surroundings
- Drugs that affect thought processes (sedatives, tranquilizers, antipsychotics)
- Drugs that increase GI/GUmotility (diuretics, laxatives, cathartics)
- Other drugs (antihypertensives)
- Use of multiple medications
- Incontinence of urine or stool
- Bandages, cast, etc., on one or both feet
- Footwear with a slippery surface
- Uses walker, cane, crutches, or wheelchair
- Uses restraint or geriatric chair
- Edema
- Postural hypotension
- Neurological disease
- Cardiovascular disease

ENVIRONMENTAL FACTORS TO CONSIDER TO REDUCE THE RISK OF ILLNESS AND INJURY

Health Care Facility Considerations

- Adequate lighting without shadows or glare
- Contrasting colors at doorways, stairs, potentially hazardous areas
- Clean, pest free, odor free
- Comfortable room temperature (72°- 75°)
- Low noise level
- Floor surface even, nonslippery
- Floor free of hazards, obstacles
- Locked cupboards or closets for chemicals, medications
- Exit doors have alarms
- Emergency call signal system in place
- Non-slip surface in bathroom, tub, and shower
- Hot water temperature regulated to 110° or according to state standards
- Protective covers on electrical outlets, heaters, fans, electrical equipment
- Protected wires
- Simple, uncluttered surroundings
- Familiar objects in room

- Designated locations for storing personal items
- Supervised smoking
- Routine environmental assessment and preventive maintenance

Home Considerations

- Telephone
- Smoke detector
- Fire extinguisher
- Adequate ventilation
- Functional refrigerator
- Minimal clutter
- Adequate lighting
- Handrail on stairs
- Floor surface even, not slippery, free of obstacles and hazards (throw rugs, electrical cords)
- Unobstructed doorways
- Doors and entryways to stairs painted a contrasting color from walls
- Non-slip surface in bathroom, tub, and shower
- Hot water temperature regulated to 110°
- Grab bars on tub and shower, if needed
- Elevated toilet seat, if needed

- Bathroom light switch easily accessible
- Windows have screens, locks
- Doors have locks
- Adequate number of electrical outlets
- Safe, working stove
- Faucet handles easy to operate, hot on left, cold on right
- Designated area for medication storage
- Outdated medications removed
- Sturdy shelves within easy reach
- Cleaning products, pesticides, chemicals properly stored
- Halls and doorways wide enough for wheelchair passage
- Absence of steps or environmental obstacles to wheelchair use
- Ramps if needed

NUTRITIONAL ASSESSMENT

A client's nutrition affects the overall state of health. To assess nutritional status, keep a record of the 24 hour intake. Then, assess the weekly intake. After a 7 day assessment is completed, you can assess the adequacy of the diet by using the USDA Food Guide Pyramid.

Review and Assess:

History:

- Cultural background
- Ethnic and economic background
- Food restrictions (medical or religious)
- Past and present eating habits
- Food preferences
- Changes in appetite and taste

Clinical Information:

- Medical diagnosis
- Height and weight
- Recent weight loss or gain
- Problems eating related to dentures, chewing, swallowing
- Food allergies

- Food/medication interactions
- Nutritional supplements
- Patient complaints of weakness, indigestion, constipation
- Elimination pattern
- Use of laxatives
- Physical function/problems that interfere with feeding or eating

Biochemical data/Laboratory tests

- Complete blood count
- Lab profile (SMA)

Identify Nursing Diagnosis:

- Aspiration: risk for
- Constipation
- Constipation, Colonic
- Constipation, Perceived
- Diarrhea
- Nutrition: Less than Body Requirements, Altered
- Nutrition: More than Body Requirements, Altered
- Nutrition: Potential for more than Body Requirements, Altered

- Self-care deficit: Feeding
- Sensory/Perceptual Alteration: Gustatory
- Sensory/Perceptual Alteration: Olfactory
- Swallowing, Impaired

Twenty Four Hour Food Intake Form

Time	Food	Amount	Food Group

AGE RELATED NUTRITIONAL RISK FACTORS

Normal aging changes may jeopardize the client's nutritional status. These include:

- Loss of enamel on teeth, teeth in various degrees of erosion or repair, missing teeth, client edentulous

- Reduction in saliva causing less efficient mixing of food and difficulty digesting starches due to decreased salivary ptyalin

- Atrophy of oral mucosa

- Decrease in number of taste buds, may use additional salt and sugar to compensate

- Reduced thirst sensation

- Reduced hunger sensation

- Gag reflex weaker, increasing risk for aspiration

- Reduced production of digestive enzymes (pepsin, hydrochloric acid, pancreatic acid), causing ineffective digestion

- Reduced fat tolerance

- Slower peristalsis, resulting in constipation

- Less efficient cholesterol regulation and absorption

NORMAL ADULT BODY WEIGHT OVER AGE 51

Women: 60 inches tall=100 pounds. Add 5 pounds for each additional inch + 10% (Add 4 pounds if less than 60 inches tall).

Men: 60 inches tall=106 pounds. Add 6 pounds for each additional inch + 10%. (Add 5 pounds if less than 60 inches tall).

	Sedentary	Moderately Active
Weight maintenance	30 calories/kg (2.2 pounds)	35 calories/kg (2.2 pounds)
Weight gain	35 calories/kg (2.2 pounds)	40 calories/kg (2.2 pounds)
Weight loss	20-25 calories/kg (2.2 pounds)	30 calories/kg (2.2 pounds)

Weight Range Calculations

Height	Weight Range	Calories required for gain	Height	Weight Range	Calories required for gain
WOMEN			MEN		
56"	79-92	1336	58"	86-105	1511
57"	79-97	1400	59"	90-111	1607
58"	81-101	1463	60"	95-117	1686
59"	87-106	1527	61"	101-123	1792
60"	90-110	1590	62"	106-130	1877
61"	95-115	1670	63"	112-136	1973
62"	99-121	1750	64"	117-143	2068
63"	104-126	1830	65"	122-150	2164
64"	108-132	1909	66"	128-156	2259
65"	113-137	1989	67"	133-163	2355
66"	117-143	2068	68"	139-169	2450
67"	122-148	2148	69"	144-176	2545
68"	126-154	2227	70"	149-183	2641
69"	131-159	2306	71"	155-189	2736
70"	135-165	2386	72"	160-196	2832
71"	140-170	2466	73"	166-202	2927
72"	144-176	2545	74"	171-209	3023
73"	148-180	2625	75"	176-216	3118
74"	153-187	2705	76"	182-222	3214
			77"	187-229	3309
			78"	193-235	3405

USDA FOOD GUIDE PYRAMID

A Guide to Daily Food Choices

The Pyramid is an outline of what to eat each day. It's not a rigid prescription, but a general guide that lets you choose a healthful diet that's right for you. The Pyramid calls for eating a variety of foods to get the nutrients you need and at the same time the right amount of calories to maintain a healthy weight.

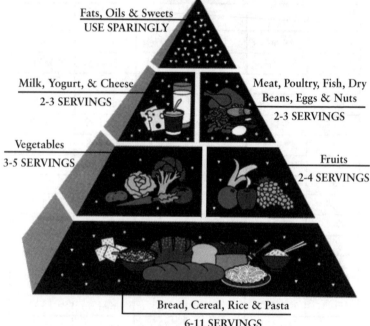

Fats, Oils & Sweets
USE SPARINGLY

Milk, Yogurt, & Cheese
2-3 SERVINGS

Meat, Poultry, Fish, Dry Beans, Eggs & Nuts
2-3 SERVINGS

Vegetables
3-5 SERVINGS

Fruits
2-4 SERVINGS

Bread, Cereal, Rice & Pasta
6-11 SERVINGS

The FOOD GUIDE PYRAMID emphasizes foods from the five food groups shown in three lower sections of the Pyramid.

Each of these food groups provides some, but not all, of the nutrients you need. Foods in one group can't replace those in another. No one food group is more important than another– for good health, you need them all.

Source: U.S. DEPARTMENT OF AGRICULTURE and the U.S. DEPARTMENT OF HEALTH AND HUMAN SERVICES

Provided by: the Education Department of the NATIONAL LIVE STOCK AND MEAT BOARD

Food Group	# of Servings per day	What constitutes a serving
Bread, cereal, rice, pasta	6-11	• 1 slice bread • 1 tortilla • 1/3 cup cooked rice, pasta, or cereal • 1 ounce ready to eat cereal • 1/2 hamburger bun, bagel, or english muffin • 3-4 plain crackers • 1 4-inch pancake • large croissant • medium doughnut or danish • 1/16 cake • 2 cookies (medium) • 1/12 pie (2 crust, 8 inch)
Vegetable	3-5	• 1/2 cup chopped raw or cooked vegetables • 1 cup raw, leafy vegetables • 3/4 cup vegetable juice • 1/2 cup scalloped potatoes • 1/2 cup potato salad • 10 french fries
Fruit	2-4	• 1 piece fruit or melon wedge • 3/4 cup fruit juice • 1/2 cup chopped, cooked, or canned fruit • 1/4 cup dried fruit
Milk, Yogurt, Cheese	2-3	• 1 cup milk or yogurt • 1-1/2 ounces natural cheese • 2 ounces process cheese • 1-1/2 cups ice cream or ice milk • 1 cup frozen yogurt

ASSESSMENT

Continued...

Food Group	# of Servings per day	What constitutes a serving
Meat, poultry, fish, dry beans, eggs, and nuts	2-3	• 2-1/2 to 3 ounces cooked lean beef, pork, lamb, veal, poultry or fish • 1/2 cup cooked beans=1 ounce meat • 1 egg=1 ounce meat • 2 tablespoons peanut butter= 1 ounce meat • 1/3 cup nuts = 1 ounce meat
Fats, Oils, Sweets	Use sparingly	Use sparingly
Calculating Mixed Foods		
Estimate the food group servings of the main ingredients. For example, a large piece of sausage pizza would count in the bread group (crust), the milk group (cheese), the meat group (sausage), and the vegetable group (tomato sauce). A helping of beef stew would count in the meat and vegetable group.		

RECOMMENDED DIETARY ALLOWANCES FOR ADULTS OVER AGE 50

	Men	Women
Calories age 50-76	2400	1800
Calories over age 76	2050	1600
Protein (g)	56	44
Vitamin A (µg RE)	1000	800
Vitamin D (µg)	5	5
Vitamin C (mg)	60	60
Thiamine (mg)	1.2	1
Riboflavin (mg)	1.4	1.2
Niacin (mg NE3)	16	13
Vitamin B6 (mg)	2.2	2
Folicin (µg)	400	400
Vitamin B12 (µg)	3	3
Calcium (mg)	800	800
Phosphorus (mg)	800	800
Magnesium (mg)	350	300
Iron (mg)	10	10
Zinc (mg)	15	15
Iodine (µg)	150	150

FOOD & DRUG INTERACTIONS

Some foods and drugs can alter the body's ability to utilize each other, causing serious side effects. Interactions will vary according to dosage, age, sex, and overall health. Common food-drug interactions are listed below.

- **Acetaminophen**-can cause toxicity if taken with more than 500 mg of vitamin C supplement daily.

- **Allopurinol**-causes decreased iron absorption.

- **Aluminum antacids**-deplete phosphate and calcium

- **Antacids (as a calcium supplement)**-avoid foods high in fiber (such as whole grains or dark, green vegetables) and oxalates (tea), which bind with the calcium and decrease absorption.

- **Antibiotics**- certain antibiotics (erythromycin, penicillin, ampicillin, and cloxacillin) should not be mixed with acidic foods, such as coffee, citrus fruits, and tomatoes because the acid interferes with absorption.

- **Anticoagulants**- a high consumption of foods high in vitamin K (spinach, cauliflower, asparagus, cabbage, potatoes, vegetable oil, brussel sprouts, egg yolk)leads to a decreased effectiveness of anticoagulant as well as increased clot formation; avoid onions, garlic, and vitamin E because they can increase the drug's effect and lead to bleeding.

- **Antihistamines**-may have prolonged effect if large amounts of alkaline foods are ingested (milk, cream, alcohol, etc.); antihistamines combined with alcohol cause drowsiness and slowed reactions.

- **Anti-HIVdrugs**-interact with many different foods, drugs, and herbal remedies; check each drug specifically for interactions.

- **Antihypertensives**-sodium reduces effectiveness.

- **Anti-infectives:**

  - **Methenamine** - cranberries, plums, prunes and their juices improve action of this drug. Avoid citrus fruits and citrus juices; eat foods with protein, but avoid dairy products.

  - **Metronidazole** - alcohol may cause stomach pain, nausea, vomiting, headache, flushing of face.

  - **Penicillins** - amoxicillin and bacampicillin may be taken with food; however, absorption of other types of penicillins is reduced when taken with food.

- **Sulfa Drugs**-may cause nausea when combined with alcohol.

- **Tetracyclines**-should not be taken within two hours of eating dairy products such as milk, yogurt or cheese, or taking calcium or iron supplements.

- **Anti-inflammatory agents**-causes stomach irritation when taken with alcohol or fruit juice; take with food or milk.

- **Aspirin**-large amounts (in excess of 12 daily) can cause vitamin C deficiency, as well as gastrointestinal bleeding and thiamine deficiency.

- **Bronchodilators**-cause central nervous system stimulation when combined with caffeine.

- **Calcium carbonate antacids**-cause deficiencies of iron, thiamine, folacin, phosphate.

- **Calcium supplements**-cause hypercalcemia when combined with large doses of vitamin D; absorption of calcium supplements decreased by foods rich in oxalate (spinach, rhubarb, celery), phytic acid (oatmeal and other grains), and phosphorus (chocolate, peanut butter, dried fruit).

- **Cigarettes-** may diminish the effectiveness of medication or create added hazards with certain medications.

- **Colchichine-**decreased effectiveness if combined with caffeine; some herbal teas contain phenylbutazone, which increases uric acid level.

- **Corticosteroids-** causes stomach irritation when combined with alcohol; fluid retention with high sodium foods.

- **Dicumerol-**effectiveness decreased with foods rich in vitamin K (spinach, cabbage, broccoli)

- **Digitalis-**may cause zinc, thiamine, and magnesium deficiencies.

- **Diuretics-** salty foods and natural black licorice increase losses of potassium and magnesium; large doses of vitamin D can cause blood pressure elevation.

- **Furosemide-**increases excretion of zinc, potassium, calcium, and magnesium.

- **Grapefruit juice-**may cause drug to be absorbed more rapidly; check for drug specific contraindications before using, particularly with calcium channel blockers and anti-HIV agents.

- **Hydralazine-**may cause vitamin B12 deficiency.

- **Iron supplements**-absorption increased by vitamin C, decreased by antacids.

- **Laxatives**-dairy foods containing calcium can decrease absorption.

- **Levodopa**-high protein diet reduces effectiveness; may cause deficiencies of B6, B12, potassium, and folacin.

- **Lithium Carbonate** -requires increased fluids; follow fluid intake instructions carefully; close monitoring of fluid balance and lithium levels required.

- **MAO Inhibitors** -very dangerous and potentially fatal; interaction can occur with foods containing tyramine, a chemical in alcoholic beverages (particularly wine), and in many foods such as hard cheeses, chocolate, beef or chicken livers.

- **Magnesium antacids**-may deplete phosphorus and calcium.

- **Mineral oil**-decreases absorption of vitamins A, D, and K.

- **Narcotic analgesics**-alcohol increases sedative effect; take with food to avoid stomach upset.

- **Phenobarbital**-decreased absorption of B6, B12, folic acid; increases breakdown of vitamins D and K.

- **Phenylbutazone**-inhibits iodine absorption.

- **Phenytoin**-reduces absorption of folacin, increases breakdown of vitamins D and K.

- **Potassium supplements**-dairy products decrease absorption.

- **Probenecid**-decreased effectiveness if coffee, tea, cola products ingested.

- **Psychotropic drugs**-interacts in a dangerous manner with alcohol; avoid alcohol completely if using.

- **Sedatives/hypnotics** and alcohol interact in a dangerous manner; avoid alcohol completely if using.

- **Spironolactone**-increases excretion of calcium; decreases excretion of potassium with the potential for causing toxicity.

- **Theophylline**-high carbohydrate diet reduces effectiveness.

- **Thiazides**-increases excretion of potassium, magnesium, calcium, zinc; can cause increased blood glucose level.

- **Thioridazine**-high alkaline diet delays excretion

- **Vasodilators**-sodium ingestion reduces effectiveness of vasodilator.

GERIATRIC LABORATORY VALUES

Blood Chemistry

Test	Age Related Variation	Normal Values
Albumin-Male sex	50-60	3.7-5.1 g/dl
	60-70	3.5-4.9 g/dl
	70-99	3.4-4.7 g/dl
Albumin-Female sex	50-60	3.7-5.1 g/dl
	60-70	3.6-4.9 g/dl
	70-99	3.4-4.7 g/dl
Bicarbonate		24-32 mEq/L
Bilirubin, total		0.1-1.0 mg/dl
Calcium		8.8-10.3 mg/dl
Chloride		95-105 mEq/L
Cholesterol, total		150-265 mg/dl
Creatinine		0.6-1.2 mg/dl
Fibrinogen		200-400 mg/dl
Glucose		70-110 mg/dl
HDL		80-310 mg/100 ml
Iodine (protein bound)		4-8μg/dl

Test	Age Related Variation	Normal Values
Iron (Fe)		Male 76-198 µg/100 ml Female 60-170 µg/100 ml
LDH		45-90 U/L
Lead		<40 µg/dl
Lipids, total		400-850 mg/dl
PCO2		22-28 mEq/L
pH		7.35-7.45
Phosphatase, acid		0-3 units/dl
Phosphatase, alkaline		30-120 units/L
Potassium		3.5-5.5 mEq/L
Protein, globulin		2.3-3.5 g/dl
Protein, total	51-61 61-71 71-99	5.9-8.0 g/dl 5.8-7.9 g/dl 5.7-7.8 g/dl
SGOT-		40 U/L
Sodium		135-145 mEq/L
Triglycerides	49-150	10-190 mg/dl
Urea Nitrogen		10-20 mg/dl
Uric Acid		Male 3.9-7.8 mg/100 ml Female 2.4-5.1 mg/100 ml

Hematology

Test	Normal Values
Hematocrit	Male 39-49% Female 33-43%
Hemoglobin	Male 13-18 g/dl Female 12-16 g/dl
Sedimentation rate	Male <20 mm/hr Female <30 mm/hr
Red blood cells	Male 4,300,000-5,900,000/mm3 Female 3,500,000-5,000,000/mm3
White blood cells	3200-9800/mm3
Neutrophils	50-70% of white blood count
Eosinophils	1-4% of white blood count
Basophils	0-1% of white blood count
Lymphoctytes	20%-40% of white blood count
Monocytes	0-6% of white blood count
Platelets	50,000-350,000/mm3
Prothrombin time	11-15 seconds

DRUG

ADMINISTRATION

DRUG ADMINISTRATION

PRINCIPLES GUIDING DRUG THERAPY IN THE ELDERLY

1. Manage medical conditions without drugs whenever possible.

2. When drug therapy is necessary, use the least number of drugs in the lowest possible dosage to manage the problem.

3. Evaluate the elderly carefully for underlying conditions that may affect or be affected by drug therapy.

4. Obtain an accurate drug history, including prescription and nonprescription drugs, vitamins, and herbs. Monitor for interactions.

5. In drugs that are excreted through the kidneys, adjust dosages using formulas that allow for age related decline.

6. Begin drug therapy with small doses and gradually increase until desired therapeutic effect is obtained.

7. Individualize the drug regimen to the client. When adding a new drug, evaluate the present regimen and remove another drug whenever possible.

8. Interpret serum levels of drugs in light of alterations in plasma protein binding.

9. Use drugs eliminated by hepatic metabolism with caution; hepatic function may be difficult to evaluate in the absence of liver disease.

10. Interview a collateral source to obtain information on the client's drug response. Ask if the client appears different since the new drug was added.

11. Monitor the client carefully for side effects and signs of toxicity.

CONDITIONS CAUSED BY GERIATRIC DRUG THERAPY

Adrenal Insufficiency	Corticosteroids
Bleeding/hemorrhage	Aspirin, NSAIDS, heparin, indomethacin, phenylbuta-zone, warfarin, Vitamin E (megadoses)
Bronchospasm	Iron (parenteral), propanolol
Candida infection	Aminoglycosides, beclomethasone (inhalation), chloramphenicol, tetracyclines
Cardiac failure	Disopyramide, guanethidine, lidocaine, propanolol

Cataracts	Corticosteroids
Colitis	Clindamycin, chloramphenicol, tetracyclines
Confusion	Alcohol, amantadine, amitriptyline, antidepressants, antidiabetic drugs, anti-parkinson agents, antipsychotics, atropine-like drugs, benzodiazepines, chlordiazepoxide, cimetidine, clonidine, diazepam, digitalis, flurazepam, glycosides, diphenhydramine, ephedrine, hydrochlorothiazide, hypnotics, indomethacin, lidocaine, methyldopa, neuroleptics, opiate narcotic analgesics, phenytoin, propanolol, propoxyphene, quinidine, reserpine, sedatives
Conjunctivitis	Hydralazine and drugs topically applied to eyes
Constipation	Aluminum hydroxide, atropine-like drugs, calcium

	carbonate, cimetidine, diuretics, iron (oral preparations), MAOIs, narcotic analgesics, verapamil
Convulsions	Haloperidol, iron (parenteral), lidocaine, lithium, MAOIs, penicillin (megadose), theophylline
Cushing's disease	Corticosteroids
Deafness	Aminoglycosides, aspirin, erythromycin, furosemide, quinidine
Delirium	Acyclovir, aminocaproic acid, amphotericin B, anticonvulsants, anticholinergic agents, antihistamines, benzodiazepines, captopril, cephalosporins, cimetidine, ciprofloxacin, clonidine, corticosteroids, digitalis, imipenemcilastatin, ketamine, ketoconazole, lidocaine, methyldopa, metoclopramide, metronidazole, narcotic analgesics, nifedipine, nitroprusside sodium, NSAIDs, penicillin, pro-

	cainamide, propranolol, quinidine sulfate, ranitidine, theophylline, trimethoprim-sulfamethoxazole
Depression	Baclofen, benzodiazepines, beta blockers, cimetidine, clonidine, corticosteroids, disulfiram, ethambutol, guanethidine, levodopa, metaclopramide, methyl-dopa, neuroleptics, propanolol, ranitidine, reser-pine, sulfonamides, thiazide diuretics
Diarrhea	Ampicillin, benzodiazepines, clindamycin, chloramphini-col, digitalis glycosides, disopyramide, guanethidine, iron (oral), KCL, laxatives, lithium, magnesium, spirono-lactone, tetracyclines, thyroid hormones, Vitamin C (megadoses)
Dysrhythmias	Adrenergic agonists, digitalis glycosides, levodopa, pro-cainamide, quinidine, theo-

	phylline, thyroid hormones, tricyclic antidepressants
Edema	Antihypertensive agents, corticosteroids, estrogens, lithium, nifedipine, phenylbutazone, sodium salts, tricyclic antidepressants
Enterocolitis, staphylococcal	Chloramphenicol, tetracyclines
Exfoliative dermatitis	Chlorpropamide, phenobarbital, phenytoin, sulfonamides
Extrapyramidal syndromes	Amoxapine, haloperidol, methyldopa, metoclopramide, neuroleptics, phenothiazines, reserpine
Galactorrhea	Cimetidine, haloperidol, methyldopa, phenothiazines
Gingival hyperplasia	Vitamin A (megadoses)
Glaucoma	Corticosteroids (opthalmic preparations), drugs possessing atropine-like activity
Goiter/hypothyroidism	Lithium, saturated solution of potassium iodide, sulfonamides
Gout	Furosemide, thiazide diuretics, Vitamin C (megadoses)

Gynecomastia	Cimetidine, diazepam, digitalis glycosides, haloperidol, phenothiazines, spironolactone
Hallucinations	Alcohol, amantadine, digitalis glycosides, ephedrine, haloperidol, levodopa, MAOIs, pentazocine, phenytoin, procainamide, propanolol
Hirsutism	Corticosteroids, minoxidil, phenytoin, spironolactone
Hyperglycemia	Corticosteroids, estrogens, furosemide, sympathomimetic amines, thiazide diuretics
Hypoglycemia	Alcohol, chloramphenicol, chlorpropamide (prolonged), fluoxetine, fluconazole, insulin, itraconazole, ketaconazole, metronidazole, propanolol, salicylates, sulfonylureas
Hypotension	Amitriptyline, antidepressants, antiemetics, antihypertensives, benzodiazepines, beta blockers, calcium channel blockers, diphenhy-

	dramine, diuretics, iron (parenteral), levodopa, lithium, MAOIs, meprobamate, metoclopramide, neuroleptics, procainamide, quinidine, theophylline, vasodilators
Hypotension, postural	Clonidine, guanethidine, haloperidol, levodopa, MAOIs, methyldopa, narcotic analgesics, nitroglycerin, phenothiazines, prazosin, reserpine, tricyclic antidepressants
Involuntary movements	Levodopa, phenothiazines
Liver dysfunction	Acetaminophen, alcohol, erythromycin estolate, haloperidol, methyldopa, phenothiazines, phenylbutazone, phenytoin, sulfonamides, sulfonylureas, tetracyclines, thiazide diuretics, Vitamin A (megadoses)
Lymphadenopathy	Iron (parenteral), primidone
Mobility impairment	Corticosteroids, heparin, lithium, phenytoin

Neuropathy, peripheral	Hydralazine, isocarboxazid, isoniazid, metronidazole, phenytoin
Nystagmus	Phenobarbital, phenytoin, primidone
Osteomalacia	Aluminum hydroxide, phenobarbital, phenytoin, primidone
Osteoporosis	Corticosteroids, heparin, thyroid hormones, vitamin D (megadoses)
Peptic ulcer	Alcohol, aspirin, caffeine, chloral hydrate, corticosteroids, nonsteroidal anti-inflammatory agents, reserpine, tobacco
Photosensitivity	Haloperidol, sulfonamides, tetracyclines, thiazide diuretics
Pneumonitis	Mineral oil
Porphyria	Barbiturates
Psychosis	Amphetamines, corticosteroids, levodopa, primidone, procainamide, quinidine, tricyclic antidepressants

Renal dysfunction	Aminoglycosides, cephalosporins, furosemide, phenylbutazone, sulfonamides, tetracyclines, thiazide diuretics, vitamin C (megadoses)
Renal stones	Aluminum hydroxide, calcium carbonate, magnesium trisilicate, vitamin C (megadoses), vitamin D (megadoses)
Stevens-Johnson syndrome	Phenylbutazone, phenytoin, sulfonamides
Systemic lupus erythematosis	Hydralazine, phenylbutazone, phenytoin, procainamide, sulfonamides
Thrombophlebitis	IV administration of cephalosporins, clindamycin, erythromycin, phenytoin, tetracyclines
Tremor	Antihistamines, hydralazine, lithium, MAOIs, tricyclic antidepressants
Unstable gait/falls	Amitriptyline, antiemetics, benzodiazepines, chlordiazepoxide, diazepam, diphenhydramine, flurazepam, over the counter

	cold remedies
Urinary retention	Amitriptyline, antiemetics, diphenhydramine
Vertigo	Aminoglycosides, aspirin, benzodiazepines, ethacrynic acid, furosemide, haloperidol, indomethacin, MAOIs, methyldopa, minocycline, phenytoin, primidone
Visual dysfunction	Amitriptyline, corticosteroids, drugs with atropine-like activity, digitalis glycosides, over the counter cold remedies, phenothiazines, phenylbutazone, phenytoin, quinidine, vitamin E (megadoses)

Blood Dyscrasias

Agranulocytosis	Antihistamines, benzodiazepines, clindamycin, phenothiazines, phenytoin, procainamide, sulfonamides, sulfonylureas, tricyclic antidepressants

Aplastic anemia	Chloramphenicol, hydralzaine, phenylbutazone, phenytoin, sulfonylureas, thiazide diuretics
Eosinophilia	Chloral hydrate, erythromycin, phenothiazines
Hemolytic anemia	Methyldopa, sulfonamides, sulfonylureas
Leukocytosis	Haloperidol, lithium, phenothiazines, tetracyclines
Leukopenia	Antihistamines, chloral hydrate, chloramphenicol, haloperidol, phenytoin, primidone
Megaloblastic anemia	Phenobarbital, phenytoin, primidone, triamterene
Neutropenia	Indomethacin, phenytoin
Reticulocytopenia	Chloramphenicol
Thrombocytopenia	Clindamycin, chloramphenicol, heparin, indomethacin, phenytoin, primidone, quinidine, sulfonamides, tetracyclines

MEDICATIONS THAT MAY CAUSE COGNITIVE IMPAIRMENT

Please note: These medications are listed as examples only. New medications appear regularly. Many compounds contain one or more active ingredients.

Type of medication and generic name

Antiarrhythmic agents: disopyramide, quinidine, tocainide

Antihistamines/decongestants: phenylpropanolamine, diphenhydramine, chlorpheniramine brompheniramine, pseudoephedrine

Antibiotics: cephalexin, cephalothin, ciprofloxacin, metronidazole, ofloxacin

Anticholinergic agents: benztropine, homatropine, scopolamine, trihexyphenidyl

Anticonvulsants: carbamazepine, phenytoin, valproic acid

Antidepressants: amitryptyline, imipramine, desipramine, fluoxetine

Antiemetics: hydroxyzine, metoclopramide, prochlor-perazine, promethazine

Antihypertensive agents: atenolol, methyldopa, meto-prolol, nifedipine, propranolol, prazosin, verapamil

Antimanic agents: lithium

Antineoplastic agents: chlorambucil, cytosine arabinoside, interleukin-2

Anti-Parkinsonian agents: bromocryptine, levodopa, pergolide

Cardiotonic agents: digoxin

Corticosteroids: hydrocortisone, prednisone

H2 receptor antagonists: cimetidine, ranitidine

Immunosuppressive agents: cyclosporine, interferon

Muscle relaxants: baclofen, cyclobenzaprine, methocarbamol

Narcotic analgesics: codeine, hydrocodone, oxycodone, meperidine, propoxyphene

Nonsteroidal anti-inflammatory agents: aspirin, ibuprofen, indomethacin, naproxen, sulindac

Radiocontrast agents: metrizamide, iothalamate, iohexol

Sedatives: alprazolam, diazepam, lorazepam, phenobarbital, butabarbital, chloral hydrate

RECOMMENDED MEDICATION ORIENTED LABORATORY TESTS FOR LONG TERM DRUG THERAPY

Medication	Test	Frequency	Purpose
Ace inhibitors	Electrolytes/CBC	Q 3 months	Monitor hyper-kalemia/blood dyscrasias
Allopurinol	BUN/Serum creatinine	Q 6 months Q 6 months	Monitor effectiveness Monitor renal function
Amino-glycosides	BUN/Serum creatinine	Q 3 days	Monitor renal function
Anti-infectives (maintenance treatment)	Urinalysis	Within 30 days	Monitor effectiveness
Anticoagulants	CBC	Q 3 months	Anemia/Blood loss
Anticonvulsants	Drug level	Q 3 months	Monitor thera-peutic range. Drug levels as needed for signs of toxicity or subtherapeutic dosing.
Butazolidin	CBC	Within 30 days	Blood dyscrasias
Chronic UTI Anti-infectives	Urinalysis	Within 30 days	Monitor effectiveness
Corticosteroids	Electrolytes	Annually	Monitor for imbalance
Digoxin with diuretic	K+	Within 30 days Q 6 months	Monitor for imbalance
Digoxin Digitoxin	Drug Level BUN/Serum Creatinine	Q 6 months Q 6 months	Monitor toxicity Monitor renal function

Continued…

Medication	Test	Frequency	Purpose
Diuretics	K+ (electrolytes) K+/MG/CA BUN/Serum Creatinine	Within 30 days Q 3 months Q 3 months	Monitor for imbalance Monitor for imbalance Monitor renal function
Diuretic K+ wasting without K+ supplement	Electrolytes	Q 2 months	Monitor for imbalance
Folic Acid/ B-12	CBC/Indices CBC/Indices/ Vitamin Level	Within 30 days Q 6 months	Monitor effectiveness
Heparin	PTT	Q 1 month	Monitor therapy range
Insulin and Oral Hypoglycemics	FBS	Q 2 months	Monitor diabetic control
Insulin	HbA1c	Q 6 months	Monitor diabetic control
Iron Supplement	CBC/Indices CBC/Indices/ Iron Level/ TIBC	Within 30 days Q 6 months	Monitor effectiveness Monitor effectiveness
Lithium	Drug Level Na+/K (Electrolytes)	Q 1 month Q 2 months	Monitor therapy/toxicity Monitor imbalance
Mandelamine /Hiprex	Urine pH	Within 30 days Q 1 month	Monitor effectiveness

Continued...

Medication	Test	Frequency	Purpose
Nitrofurantoin	BUN/Serum Creatinine	Within 30 days Q 6 months	Monitor renal function
NSAIDs	CBC BUN/Serum Creatinine/K+ SGOT	Q 3 months Q 3 months Q 3 months	Anemia/GI Blood Loss Monitor renal function Monitor liver function
Antipsychotics	SGOT	Annually	Monitor liver function
Septra/Bactrim	CBC/Indices/Platelets	Q 6 months	Monitor blood dyscrasias
Thyroid products	Thyroid panel/TSH/T4	Q 6 months	Monitor dosage. Drug levels as needed for signs of toxicity or subtherapeutic dosing.
L-Thyroxine	T4/TSH	Q 6 months	Monitor dosage.
Warfarin	Prothrombin time	Q 1 months	Monitor therapy range

Note: Yearly physical should include electrolytes, U/A, CBC with differential, SGOT, thyroid panel, TB screening. The frequency of laboratory monitoring will depend upon the client's overall condition, signs and symptoms of toxicity or treatment failure, and will require clinical judgment.

RISK FACTORS FOR SELF ADMINISTRATION OF MEDICATION

- Visual impairment
- Hearing impairment
- Cognitive impairment
- Inability to read (illiterate)
- Arthritis or weakness in hands
- History of non-compliance with medications
- History of inappropriate self medication
- Use of multiple medications
- Presence of discontinued or expired medications
- Presence of borrowed medications
- Lack of knowledge regarding medications
- Use of multiple medications (polypharmacy)
- Seeing multiple physicians and not giving each physician a complete drug history
- Using multiple pharmacies
- Lack of financial resources to purchase medications

INFECTION

CONTROL

Infection Control

MODE OF TRANSMISSION OF PATHOGENS

According to the Centers for Disease Control, there are five methods in which pathogens can be transferred to others:

1. Contact transmission
   - The most frequent method of transmission
   - Two subgroups:
     - Direct contact-direct body surface to body surface contact and physical transfer of microorganisms
     - Indirect contact-contact of a susceptible host with a contaminated intermediate object, usually inanimate

2. Droplet transmission
   - Respiratory secretions generated from coughing, sneezing, talking, laughing, and singing and in the performance of some procedures, such as suctioning and bronchoscopy.
   - Droplets usually remain within 3 feet of the client and are deposited on the host's conjunctiva, nasal mucosa, or mouth. These droplets do not remain suspended in the air.

3. Airborne transmission
   - Dissemination of respiratory droplets that are tiny and light weight; these droplets remain

suspended in the air for long periods and travel long distances on dust, air currents, and moisture.

- Inhaled by the susceptible host

4. Common Vehicle Transmission
   - Transmitted by contaminated items such as food, water, medications, devices, and equipment.

5. Vector-borne Transmission
   - Transmitted by insects and vermin

STANDARD PRECAUTIONS

In 1996, the Centers for Disease Control and Prevention published a new set of guidelines to prevent the transmission of disease. These precautions were designed to replace universal precautions and body substance isolation and are used in the care of all clients, regardless of disease status.

Standard precautions apply to blood, all body fluids (except sweat), secretions, excretions, mucous membranes, and nonintact skin.

- Handwashing
    - Should be done before and after each client contact
    - Should be done after contact with blood, body fluids, secretions, excretions, and

equipment (or articles contaminated by them)
- Should be done after gloves are removed
- A standard nonantimicrobial soap is used for routine handwashing
- Antimicrobial soap or a waterless antiseptic agent is used in control of outbreaks or hyperendemic infections

• Gloves:
- Provide a barrier and prevent gross contamination of the hands when touching blood, body fluids, secretions, excretions, mucous membranes, and nonintact skin
- Reduce the likelihood that pathogens will be present on hands of personnel during invasive or other patient care procedures involving touching mucous membranes, nonintact skin, or body cavities
- Reduce the likelihood that pathogens from another client or fomite will be transmitted from the hands of the personnel to a client
- Wearing gloves does not replace the need for handwashing because gloves can have microscopic defects or may be torn during use. Hands can become contaminated during glove removal

- Gloves are changed if they come into contact with high concentrations of infective material (e.g. fecal matter), and immediately before contact with mucous membranes or nonintact skin
- It may be necessary to change gloves and wash hands several times during the care of one client to prevent cross contamination between body sites

- Masks, Respiratory Protection, Eye Protection and Face Shields
  - Worn during procedures, care activities, and equipment reprocessing likely to generate splashes or sprays of blood, body fluids, secretions, or excretions

- Gowns and Protective Apparel
  - Worn to prevent contamination of clothing and protect skin from blood and body fluid exposures
  - Gowns should be specially treated to make them impermeable to liquids
  - Leg covers, boots, or shoe covers provide greater protection when large quantities of infective material are present or splashes are anticipated

– Protective apparel is selected according to the type of procedure and is removed as promptly as possible after the procedure to avoid environmental contamination. Hands are washed after apparel is removed

- Sharps
  – Needles are not recapped, bent, broken, or cut; if recapping is necessary, the one hand scoop method is used

- Resuscitation
  – Mouthpieces, resuscitation bags, and other ventilation devices are used to minimize the risk of pathogen exposure through mouth to mouth contact

- Client Care Equipment and Other Articles
  – Used sharps are placed in puncture resistant containers as close to the site of use as practical
  – Other equipment is single bagged; double bagging is used only if the outside of the original bag becomes contaminated during the bagging process
  – Contaminated, reusable equipment (e.g. equipment that normally enters sterile tissue or through which blood flows) is disinfected and sterilized after use

- Noncritical equipment (e.g. blood pressure cuff) is cleaned and disinfected after use
- Disposable equipment is handled and transported in a manner that reduces the risk of transmission of pathogens and avoids environmental contamination

• Linen and Laundry

- The risk of disease transmission is negligible if laundry is handled, transported, and laundered in a manner that avoids the transfer of microorganisms
- Single bagging is used unless the outside of the bag becomes contaminated during the bagging process

• Dishes, Glasses, Cups, and Eating Utensils

- No special precautions are required. The combination of hot water and detergent in the dishwasher is sufficient to decontaminate these items

• Routine and Terminal Cleaning

- All rooms are cleaned using the same terminal cleaning procedures unless the amount of infective organisms or environmental contamination indicates special cleaning is required. Adequate disinfection of bedside equipment and environmental surfaces is essential

Avoiding Environmental Contamination

The Centers for Disease Control and Preventions recommendations note that the health care worker should avoid environmental contamination with used personal protective equipment. This is a particularly great concern with contaminated gloves. Removing one glove before touching environmental surfaces or items may be appropriate. Use the ungloved hand to open doors, turn on faucets, and handle other items. If removing a glove is not possible, holding a paper towel under the gloved hand may be an option. Use the paper towel to contact environmental surfaces.

Agency requirements vary regarding how and where contaminated gloves are disposed. Most health care agencies require glove disposal in a closed, plastic container. This may be a covered waste can or closed plastic bag. The nurse should know and follow local regulations and facility policies for glove disposal.

TRANSMISSION-BASED PRECAUTIONS

Transmission-based precautions are the second tier of the 1996 CDC recommendations. These precautions are implemented in clients who are known or suspected to be infectious. Standard precautions are always used in addition to transmission-based precautions. Four of the previously used isolation categories have been eliminated. The use of more than one transmission-based precautions category may be indicated in clients with diseases or conditions with multiple modes of transmission.

- Client Placement
    - A private room is used to prevent transmission or when the source client has poor hygiene, contaminates the environment, or cannot be expected to assist in maintaining infection control precautions.
    - Cohorting is acceptable when two clients have the same disease, the likelihood of reinfection with the same infection is minimal, and no other co-existing infections are present. Avoid sharing a room if one client has additional infective organisms that can be spread to roommates.
- Transport of Infected Clients
    - Limit movement or transport whenever possible.
    - When transport of clients in isolation is essential:
        - Clients in airborne or droplet precautions, should wear a surgical mask when out of the room.
        - Clients in contact precautions should

have the infective secretions covered
with an impervious dressing or other
barrier.

- Personnel in the receiving area are notified in advance of the impending arrival
and are notified of precautions to use.

- The client must be informed of ways to
assist in preventing the transfer of their
infectious organisms to others.

Transmission-Based Precautions Categories

- Airborne Precautions
  - Used for diseases that are spread through
  tiny droplets in air currents
  (e.g. Tuberculosis).
  - Special air handling and ventilation in the
  room are required.
    - Negative pressure environment with 6-
    12 complete air changes per hour.
    - Exhaust from room directly ventilated
    to outside or specially filtered to prevent
    passage by microorganisms.
    - Door to the room must remain closed.
  - Personnel wear HEPA, N95, or PFR 95
  respirators when entering the room (Must
  used NIOSH approved respirator).

- No other special precautions required unless necessary to implement the principles of standard precautions.

- Droplet Precautions
    - No special air handling is required.
    - Door to the room may remain open.
    - Personnel wear surgical masks.
    - No other special precautions required unless necessary to implement the principles of standard precautions.
    - No other special precautions required unless necessary to implement the principles of standard precautions.

- Contact Precautions
    - Gloves are worn when entering the room.
        - Gloves are changed if they contact infective material.
        - Avoid contamination of environmental surfaces with gloves.
        - Gloves are removed and hands washed with an antimicrobial agent or waterless antiseptic agent before leaving the room; avoid inadvertent contamination of hands on environmental surfaces after handwashing.
    - A gown is worn if your uniform will have

substantial contact with the client, environmental surfaces, or if the client is incontinent, has diarrhea, an ostomy, or wound drainage not contained by a dressing.

- Remove the gown immediately before leaving the room and avoid inadvertent contamination of your uniform from environmental surfaces.

- No other special precautions required unless necessary to implement the principles of standard precautions.

Type and Duration of Precautions Needed for Selected Infections and Conditions

Abbreviations: type of precautions:

A	Airborne
C	Contact
D	Droplet
S	Standard; when A, C, and D are specified, also use S.

+ Duration of precautions:

CN	until off antibiotics and culture-negative;
DH	duration of hospitalization;

DI   duration of illness (with wound
lesions, DI means until they stop
draining)

U   until time specified in hours (hrs) after
initiation of effective therapy

F   see footnote number.

Infection/Condition	Type*	Duration+
Abscess		
Draining, major (1)	C	DI
Draining, minor or limited (2)	S	
Acquired immunodeficiency syndrome (3)	S	
Actinomycosis	S	
Adenovirus infection, in infants and young children	D,C	DI
Amebiasis	S	
Anthrax		
Cutaneous	S	
Pulmonary	S	
Antibiotic-associated colitis (see Clostridium difficile)		
Arthropodborne viral encephalitides (eastern, western, Venezuelan equine encephalomyelitis; St. Louis, California encephalitis)	S (4)	

Infection/Condition	Type*	Duration+
Arthropodborne viral fevers (dengue, yellow fever, Colorado tick fever)	S (4)	
Ascariasis	S	
Aspergillosis	S	
Babesiosis	S	
Blastomycosis, North American, cutaneous or pulmonary	S	
Botulism	S	
Bronchiolitis (see respiratory infections in infants and young children)		
Brucellosis (undulant, Malta, Mediterranean fever)	S	
Campylobacter gastroenteritis (see gastroenteritis)		
Candidiasis, all forms including mucocutaneous	S	
Cat-scratch fever (benign inoculation lymphoreticulosis)	S	
Cellulitis, uncontrolled drainage	C	DI
Chancroid (soft chancre)	S	
Chickenpox (varicella; see F (5) for varicella exposure)	A,C	F (5)
Chlamydia trachomatis		
Conjunctivitis	S	
Genital	S	
Respiratory	S	

Infection/Condition	Type*	Duration+
Cholera (see gastroenteritis)		
Closed-cavity infection		
Draining, limited or minor	S	
Not draining	S	
Clostridium		
C botulinum	S	
C difficile	C	DI
C perfringens		
Food poisoning	S	
Gas gangrene	S	
Coccidioidomycosis (valley fever)		
Draining lesions	S	
Pneumonia	S	
Colorado tick fever	S	
Congenital rubella	C	F (6)
Conjunctivitis		
Acute bacterial	S	
Chlamydia	S	
Gonococcal	S	
Acute viral (acute hemorrhagic)	C	DI
Coxsackievirus disease (see enteroviral infection)		
Creutzfeldt-Jakob disease	S (7)	
Croup (see respiratory infections in infants and young children		
Cryptococcosis	S	
Cryptosporidiosis (see gastroenteritis)		

Infection/Condition	Type*	Duration+
Cysticercosis	S	
Cytomegalovirus infection, neonatal or immunosuppressed	S	
Decubitus ulcer, infected		
Major (1)	C	DI
Minor or limited (2)	S	
Dengue	S (4)	
Diarrhea, acute — infective etiology suspected (see gastroenteritis)		
Diphtheria		
Cutaneous	C	CN (8)
Pharyngeal	D	CN (8)
Ebola viral hemorrhagic fever	C (9)	DI
Echinococcosis (hydatidosis)	S	
Echovirus (see enteroviral infection)		
Encephalitis or encephalomyelitis (see specific etiologic agents)		
Endometritis	S	
Enterobiasis (pinworm disease, oxyuriasis)	S	
Enterococcus species (see multidrug-resistant organisms if epidemiologically significant or vancomycin resistant)		
Enterocolitis, Clostridium difficile	C	DI

INFECTION
CONTROL

Infection/Condition	Type*	Duration+
Enteroviral infections		
Adults	S	
Infants and young children	C	DI
Epiglottitis, due to Haemophilus influenzae	D	U (24 hrs)
Epstein-Barr virus infection, including infectious mononucleosis	S	
Erythema infectiosum (also see Parvovirus B19)	S	
Escherichia coli gastroenteritis (see gastroenteritis)		
Food poisoning		
Botulism	S	
Clostridium perfringens or welchii	S	
Staphylococcal	S	
Furunculosis — staphylococcal		
Infants and young children	C	DI
Gangrene (gas gangrene)	S	
Gastroenteritis		
Campylobacter species	S (10)	
Cholera		S (10)
Clostridium difficile	C	DI
Cyptosporidium species	S (10)	
Escherichia coli		
Enterohemorrhagic O157:H7	S (10)	
Diapered or incontinent	C	DI
Other species	S (10)	

Infection/Condition	Type*	Duration+
Giardia lamblia	S (10)	
Rotavirus	S (10)	
Diapered or incontinent	C	DI
Salmonella species including S typhi)	S (10)	
Shigella species	S (10)	
Diapered or incontinent	C	DI
Vibrio parahaemolyticus	S (10)	
Viral (if not covered elsewhere)	S (10)	
Yersinia enterocolitica	S (10)	
German measles (rubella)	D	F (22)
Giardiasis (see gastroenteritis)		
Gonococcal ophthalmia neonatorum (gonorrheal opthalmia acute conjunctivitis of newborn)	S	
Gonorrhea	S	
Granuloma inguinale donovanosis, granuloma venereum)	S	
Guillain-Barre syndrome	S	
Hand, foot, and mouth disease (see enteroviral infection)		
Hantavirus pulmonary syndrome	S	
Helicobacter pylori	S	
Hemorrhagic fevers (for example, Lassa and Ebola)	C (9)	DI

Infection/Condition	Type*	Duration+
Hepatitis, viral		
Type A S		
Diapered or incontinent patients	C	F (11)
Type B — HBsAg positive	S	
Type C and other unspecified		
non-A, non-B	S	
Type E	S	
Herpangina (see enteroviral infection)		
Herpes simplex (Herpesvirus hominis)		
Encephalitis	S	
Neonatal (12) (see F (12)		
for neonatal exposure)	C	DI
Mucocutaneous, disseminated		
or primary, severe	C	DI
Mucocutaneous, recurrent		
(skin, oral, genital)	S	
Herpes zoster (varicella-zoster)		
Localized in immunocompromised		
patient, or disseminated	A,C	DI (13)
Localized in normal patient	S (13)	
Histoplasmosis	S	
HIV (see human immunodeficiency virus	S	
Hookworm disease		
(ancylostomiasis, uncinariasis)	S	
Human immunodeficiency virus		
(HIV) infection (3)	S	
Impetigo	C	U (24 hrs)

Infection/Condition	Type*	Duration+
Infectious mononucleosis	S	
Influenza	D (14)	DI
Kawasaki syndrome	S	
Lassa fever	C (9)	DI
Legionnaires' disease	S	
Leprosy	S	
Leptospirosis	S	
Lice (pediculosis)	C	U (24)
Listeriosis	S	
Lyme disease	S	
Lymphocytic choriomeningitis	S	
Lymphogranuloma venereum	S	
Malaria	S (4)	
Marburg virus disease	C (9)	DI
Measles (rubeola), all presentations	A	DI
Melioidosis, all forms	S	
Meningitis Aseptic (nonbacterial or viral meningitis {also see enteroviral infections})	S	
Bacterial, gram-negative enteric, in neonates	S	
Fungal	S	

Infection/Condition	Type*	Duration+
Meningitis (continued)		
Haemophilus influenzae, known or suspected	D	U (24 hrs)
Listeria monocytogenes	S	
Neisseria meningitidis (meningococcal) known or suspected	D	U (24 hrs)
Pneumococcal	S	
Tuberculosis (15)	S	
Other diagnosed bacterial	S	
Meningococcal pneumonia	D	U (24 hrs)
Meningococcemia (meningococcal sepsis)	D	U (24 hrs)
Molluscum contagiosum	S	
Mucormycosis	S	
Multidrug-resistant organisms, infection or colonization (16)		
Gastrointestinal	C	CN
Respiratory	C	CN
Pneumococcal	S	
Skin, wound, or burn	C	CN
Mumps (infectious parotitis	D	F (17))
Mycobacteria, nontuberculosis (atypical)		
Pulmonary	S	
Wound	S	
Mycoplasma pneumonia	D	DI
Necrotizing enterocolitis	S	

Infection/Condition	Type*	Duration+
Nocardiosis, draining lesions or other presentations	S	
Norwalk agent gastroenteritis (see viral gastroenteritis)		
Orf	S	
Parainfluenza virus infection, respiratory in infants and young children	C	DI
Parvovirus B19	D	F (18)
Pediculosis (lice)	C	U (24 hrs)
Pertussis (whooping cough)	D	F (19)
Pinworm infection	S	
Plague		
Bubonic	S	
Pneumonic	D	U (72 hrs)
Pleurodynia (see enteroviral infection)		
Pneumonia		
Adenovirus	D,C	DI
Bacterial not listed elsewhere (including gram-negative bacterial)	S	
Burkholderia cepacia in cystic fibrosis (CF) patients, including respiratory tract colonization	S (20)	
Chlamydia	S	
Fungal	S	

Infection/Condition	Type*	Duration+
Pneumonia (continued)		
Haemophilus influenzae		
Adults	S	
Infants and children (any age)	D	U (24 hrs)
Legionella	S	
Meningococcal	D	U (24 hrs)
Multidrug-resistant bacterial (see multidrug-resistant organisms)		
Mycoplasma (primary atypical pneumonia)	D	DI
Pneumococcal		
Multidrug-resistant (see multidrug-resistant organisms)		
Pneumocystis carinii	S (21)	
Pseudomonas cepacia (see Burkholderia cepacia)	S (20)	
Staphylococcus aureus	S	
Streptococcus, Group A		
Adults	S	
Infants and young children	D	U (24 hrs)
Viral		
Adults	S	
Infants and young children (see respiratory infectious disease, acute)		
Poliomyelitis	S	
Psittacosis (ornithosis)	S	

Infection/Condition	Type*	Duration+
Q fever	S	
Rabies	S	

Rat-bite fever
    (Streptobacillus moniliformis disease,
    Spirillum minus disease)
	S	

Relapsing fever	S	
Resistant bacterial infection or colonization see multidrug-resistant organisms)		

Respiratory infectious disease, acute
(if not covered elsewhere)
    Adults
    Infants and young children (3)
	
	S
	C
		
		DI

Respiratory syncytial virus infection, in infants and young children, and immunocompromised adults	C	DI
Reye's syndrome	S	
Rheumatic fever	S	

Rickettsial fevers, tickborne
    (Rocky Mountain spotted fever,
    tickborne typhus fever)
	S	

Rickettsialpox (vesicular rickettsiosis)	S	
Ringworm (dermatophytosis, dermatomycosis, tinea)	S	
Ritter's disease (staphylococcal scalded skin syndrome)	S	
Rocky Mountain spotted fever	S	

Infection/Condition	Type*	Duration+
Roseola infantum (exanthem subitum)	S	
Rotavirus infection (see gastroenteritis)		
Rubella (German measles; also see congenital rubella)	D	F (22)
Salmonellosis (see gastroenteritis)		
Scabies	C	U (24 hrs)
Scalded skin syndrome, staphylococcal (Ritter's disease)	S	
Schistosomiasis (bilharziasis)	S	
Shigellosis (see gastroenteritis)		
Sporotrichosis	S	
Spirillum minus disease (rat-bite fever)	S	
Staphylococcal disease (S aureus)	S	
Skin, wound, or burn		
Major (1)	C	DI
Minor or limited (2)	S	
Enterocolitis	S (10)	
Multidrug-resistant see multidrug-resistant organisms)		
Pneumonia	S	
Scalded skin syndrome	S	
Toxic shock syndrome	S	

Infection/Condition	Type*	Duration+
Streptobacillus moniliformis disease rat-bite fever)	S	
Streptococcal disease (group A streptococcus)		
Skin, wound, or burn		
Major (1)	C	U (24 hrs)
Minor or limited (2)	S	
Endometritis (puerperal sepsis)	S	
Pharyngitis in infants and young children	D	U (24 hrs)
Pneumonia in infants and young children	D	U (24 hrs)
Scarlet fever in infants and young children	D	U (24 hrs)
Streptococcal disease (group B streptococcus) neonatal	S	
Streptococcal disease (not group A or B) unless covered elsewhere	S	
Multidrug-resistant (see multidrug-resistant organisms)		
Strongyloidiasis	S	
Syphilis		
Skin and mucous membrane, including congenital, primary, secondary	S	
Latent (tertiary) and seropositivity without lesions	S	
Tapeworm disease		
Hymenolepis nana	S	
Taenia solium (pork)	S	
Other	S	

Infection/Condition	Type*	Duration+
Tetanus	S	
Tinea (fungus infection dermatophytosis, dermatomycosis, ringworm)	S	
Toxoplasmosis	S	
Toxic shock syndrome (staphylococcal disease)	S	
Trachoma, acute	S	
Trench mouth (Vincent's angina	S)	
Trichinosis	S	
Trichomoniasis	S	
Trichuriasis (whipworm disease)	S	
Tuberculosis		
Extrapulmonary, draining lesion (including scrofula)	S	
Extrapulmonary, meningitis (15)	S	
Pulmonary, confirmed or suspected or laryngeal disease	A	F (23)
Skin-test positive with no evidence of current pulmonary disease	S	
Tularemia		
Draining lesion	S	
Pulmonary	S	
Typhoid (Salmonella typhi) fever (see gastroenteritis)		

Infection/Condition	Type*	Duration+
Typhus, endemic and epidemic	S	
Urinary tract infection (including pyelonephritis), with or without urinary catheter	S	
Varicella (chickenpox)	A,C	F (5)
Vibrio parahaemolyticus (see gastroenteritis)		
Vincent's angina (trench mouth)	S	
Viral diseases		
Respiratory (if not covered elsewhere)		
Adults	S	
Infants and young children (see respiratory infectious disease acute)		
Whooping cough (pertussis)	D	F (19)
Wound infections		
Major (1)	C	DI
Minor or limited (2)	S	
Yersinia enterocolitica gastroenteritis (see gastroenteritis)		
Localized in immunocompromised patient, disseminated	A,C	DI (13)
Localized in normal patient	S (13)	
Zygomycosis (phycomycosis, mucormycosis)	S	
Zoster (varicella-zoster)		

(1.)   No dressing or dressing does not contain drainage adequately.

(2.)   Dressing covers and contains drainage adequately.

(3.)   Also see syndromes of conditions listed in Table 2.

(4.)   Install screens in windows and doors in
        endemic areas.

(5.)   Maintain precautions until all lesions are crusted. The average
        incubation period for varicella is 10 to 16 days, with a range of 10
        to 21 days. After exposure, use varicella zoster immune globin
        (VZIG) when appropriate, and discharge susceptible patients if
        possible. Place exposed susceptible patients on Airborne
        Precautions beginning 10 days after exposure and continuing until
        21 days after last exposure (up to 28 days if VZIG has been given).
        Susceptible persons should not enter the room of patients on
        precautions if other immune caregivers are available.

(6.)   Place infant on precautions during any admission until 1 year of
        age, unless nasopharyngeal and urine cultures are negative for virus
        after age 3 months.

(7.)   Additional special precautions are necessary for handling and
        decontamination of blood, body fluids and tissues, and contami-
        nated items from patients with confirmed or suspected disease. See
        latest College of American Pathologists (Northfield, Illinois)
        guidelines or other references.

(8.)   Until two cultures taken at least 24 hours apart are negative.

(9.)   Call state health department and CDC for specific advice about
        management of a suspected case. During the 1995 Ebola outbreak
        in Zaire, interim recommendations were published. (97) Pending a
        comprehensive review of the epidemiologic data from the outbreak
        and evaluation of the interim recommendations, the 1988
        guidelines for management of patients with suspected viral
        hemorrhagic infections (16) will be reviewed and updated if
        indicated.

(10.)   Use Contact Precautions for diapered or incontinent children 6 years of
        age for duration of illness.

(11.)   Maintain precautions in infants and children 3 years of age for duration of hospitalization; in children 3 to 14 years of age, until 2 weeks after onset of symptoms; and in others, until 1 week after onset of symptoms.

(12.)   For infants delivered vaginally or by C-section and if mother has active infection and membranes have been ruptured for more than 4 to 6 hours.

(13.)   Persons susceptible to varicella are also at risk for developing varicella when exposed to patients with herpes zoster lesions; therefore, susceptibles should not enter the room if other immune caregivers are available.

(14.)   The Guideline for Prevention of Nosocomial Pneumonia (95,96) recommends surveillance, vaccination, antiviral agents, and use of private rooms with negative air pressure as much as feasible for patients for whom influenza is suspected or diagnosed. Many hospitals encounter logistic difficulties and physical plant limitations when admitting multiple patients with suspected influenza during community outbreaks. If sufficient private rooms are unavailable, consider cohorting patients or, at the very least, avoid room sharing with high-risk patients. See Guideline for Prevention of Nosocomial Pneumonia (95,96) for additional prevention and control strategies.

(15.)   Patient should be examined for evidence of current (active) pulmonary tuberculosis. If evidence exists, additional precautions are necessary (see tuberculosis).

(16.)   Resistant bacteria judged by the infection control program, based on current state, regional, or national recommendations, to be of special nclinical and epidemiologic significance.

(17.)   For 9 days after onset of swelling.

(18.)   Maintain precautions for duration of hospitalization when chronic disease occurs in an immunodeficient patient. For patients with transient aplastic crisis or red-cell crisis, maintain precautions for 7 days.

(19.)   Maintain precautions until 5 days after patient is placed on effective therapy.

(20.)   Avoid cohorting or placement in the same room with a CF patient who is not infected or colonized with B cepacia. Persons with CF who visit or provide care and are not infected or colonized with B cepacia may elect to wear a mask when within 3 ft of a colonized or infected patient.

(21.)   Avoid placement in the same room with an immunocompromised patient.

(22.)   Until 7 days after onset of rash.

(23.)   Discontinue precautions only when TB patient is on effective therapy, is improving clinically, and has three consecutive negative sputum smears collected on different days, or TB is ruled out. Also see CDC Guidelines for Preventing the Transmission of Tuberculosis in Health-Care Facilities. (23)

TUBERCULOSIS

Tuberculosis has become a major public health problem of the 1990's. Many elderly persons were infected with the causative agent, Mycobacterium tuberculosis, decades ago. The bacteria has remained in their body for years, kept inactive by a healthy immune system. Approximately 10% of individuals previously infected with *Mycobacterium tuberculosis* will develop active tuberculosis disease.

The Centers for Disease Control and Prevention (CDC) recommends two step tuberculin testing as a method of evaluating an individual's infection status. The frequency of testing is determined by the degree of risk. Many health care agencies are routinely screening geriatric clients for tuberculosis as part of their routine physical examination. The procedure for administering and interpreting the two step tuberculin test follows.

Two-Step Tuberculin Testing

1. Inject 0.1 ml of purified protein derivative vaccine (5 tuberculin units) intradermally 4 inches below the antecubital space.

2. Observe the area 48 to 72 hours after the injection. Disregard the erythema. Using a metric rule, measure the indurated (raised) area.

3. Record the millimeters of induration. If over 10, no additional testing should be done. Refer to the physician or public health department.

If indurated area is 10 mm. diameter or less:

4. Repeat steps 1 to 3 above within 7 to 14 days.

Interpretation of Tuberculin Tests

1. A reaction of ≥ 5 mm induration is considered positive in the following:

   a. Clients with HIV infection or risk factors for HIV infection with unknown HIV status.

   b. Clients who have had recent close contact with an individual with active TB.

   c. Clients with fibrotic chest x-rays consistent with old healed TB.

2. A reaction of ≥10 mm induration is considered positive in all clients who fail to meet the above criteria but have other risk factors for TB including:

   a. HIV seronegative intravenous drug users.

   b. Clients with medical conditions known to increase the risk of progression from latent TB to active TB including silicosis, gastrectomy, jejunoileal bypass, 10% below ideal body weight, chronic renal failure, diabetes, receiving high dose corticosteroids, clients with leukemia, and those with other malignancies.

   c. Foreign born clients from high prevalence countries in Africa, Asia, Latin America and the Caribbean.

   d. Clients from low income, medically underserved populations.

   e. Residents of long-term care facilities and prisons.

   f. Individuals from high risk populations in the community as determined by the local health department.

3. A reaction of ≥15 mm induration is considered positive in individuals who do not meet any of the above criteria.

4. Recent converters are classified on the basis of induration and age:

a. ≥10 mm induration increase within a 2 year period is considered positive for persons ≤ 35 years.

b. ≥ 15 mm induration increase within a 2 year period is considered positive for persons ≥ 35 years.

c. ≥ 5 mm increase under certain circumstances (see 1 a, b, c).

Health Care Worker Screening for Tuberculosis

Risk Assessment

Analyze PPD test conversion data, number of TB cases, and other risk factors by area and occupational group

PPD test conversion rate significantly greater than areas without TB clients or than previous rate in same area

or

Cluster of PPD test conversions (Two or more PPD conversions in one area or a single occupational group that works in multiple areas over a 3 month period)

or

Evidence of client- to- client transmission

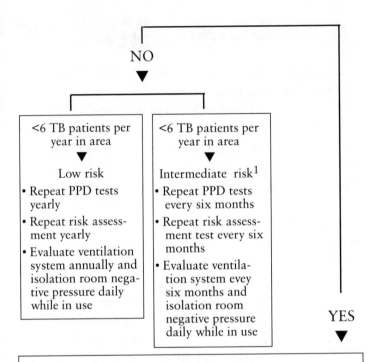

NO

<6 TB patients per year in area	<6 TB patients per year in area
▼	▼
Low risk	Intermediate risk[1]
• Repeat PPD tests yearly	• Repeat PPD tests every six months
• Repeat risk assessment yearly	• Repeat risk assessment test every six months
• Evaluate ventilation system annually and isolation room negative pressure daily while in use	• Evaluate ventilation system evey six months and isolation room negative pressure daily while in use

YES ▼

High risk
- Initiate problem evaluation
- Repeat PPD tests every 3 months
- Repeat risk assessment every 3 months and isolation room negative pressure daily while in use
- Consider supplemental engineering measures
- Maintain highest index of suspicion for potential TB patients

INFECTION CONTROL

[1]Occurance of drug resistant TB in the faculty or the community or high prevalance of HIV infection among clients or workers in the facility may warrant a higher risk rating.

HERPES ZOSTER (SHINGLES)

Herpes zoster is common in the elderly. The disorder is named from both Latin and French words for belt, or girdle. It refers to skin eruptions on the trunk.

Herpes zoster is caused by the same virus that causes chicken pox. Anyone who has had chicken pox can develop shingles later in life. There is no known prevention. Although more common in the elderly, eruptions can occur at any age. About 20 percent of the population is affected at some time during their lives. The virus remains in the nerve cells in a dormant state. If the virus awakens, shingles, or zoster, erupts on the body. The cause of the viral reactivation is unknown, although it is believed to be caused by a temporary weakeness in the immune system allowing the virus to reproduce and move along nerve fibers to the skin. Since herpes zoster commonly affects older adults, this supports the weakened immune response theory. Stress or trauma may also also trigger a zoster attack. Immune compromised individuals are more inclined to develop herpes zoster. Many of these individuals are severely affected. This high risk group includes individuals with HIV disease and AIDS, cancer, such as leukemia or lymphoma, or clients treated with chemotherapy or radiation therapy. Individuals who are taking immunosuppressants because of organ transplants are also susceptible.

Signs and Symptoms of Herpes Zoster

- Burning pain or tingling 48 hours prior to rash eruption.

- Extreme sensitivity in a specific area of the skin.

- Fever

- Headache

- Eruption of an acute, vesicular rash one to three days after the client becomes symptomatic.

- The rash is confined to one side of the body.

- The rash turns into groups of blisters that are similar in appearance to chicken pox.

- Blisters last for two to three weeks.

- Pus collects in the blisters. Gradually the blisters crust over and begin to disappear.

- Some individuals develop swelling of regional lymph nodes.

- Pain may be persistent, and follows the course of a nerve. Having pain without blisters or blisters without pain is uncommon.

- The pain of herpes zoster is severe and frequently requires narcotic analgesics.

- Herpes zoster is most common on the trunk and buttocks. However, they can also appear on the face. Blisters on the tip of the nose may be an indication of eye involvement. If blisters appear on the nose or near the eyes, refer the client to an opthalmologist immediately.

Complications of Herpes Zoster

- Post-herpetic neuralgia is a condition in which constant, severe pain or periods of intermittent pain continue after the skin heals. The neuralgia can last for years and is more common in those over 70. Some physicians believe that treating an active outbreak with narcotic analgesics will prevent this complication.

- Secondary bacterial infection of the lesions, which can delay healing. If healing progresses normally, then pain and redness recur, refer to a dermatologist for antibiotic therapy.

- Widespread dissemination of the zoster lesions occurs in two to five percent of clients, most commonly those with weakened immune systems and underlying disorders. Internal organs may also be affected.

- Anesthesia

- Scarring

- Facial or other nerve paralysis

- Encephalitis

- Zoster opthalmicus results in visual impairment.

Diagnosis

- Appearance of painful blisters on one side of the body.

- Cells can be examined microscopically, as can fluid from the lesions.

- Tzanck smear may be positive, particularly in early lesions.

Mode of Transmission

- The virus can be transmitted to others, but those infected will develop chicken pox.

- Herpes zoster is much less contagious than chicken pox.

- The virus is transmitted through drainage from the lesions.

- The client is no longer infectious when the lesions dry and crust over.

- Individuals who are immunocompromised and those who have not had chicken pox should avoid contact with the client.

- Standard precautions are adequate to prevent transmission.

- Airborne and contact precautions are used for localized zoster in immunocompromised clients, or widely disseminated zoster.

Treatment

- In most people, the condition clears on its own in a few weeks and may not recur.

- Adequate hydration

- Monitor renal function in high risk or impaired clients

- Analgesics

- Cool compresses

- Calamine lotion applied directly to lesions may be helpful

- Antiviral drugs such as acyclovir and famciclovir do not eliminate the virus, but do prevent it from replicating. Antivirals are available in oral and topical preparations. The preparations are most effective if given early in the illness. The drugs do not prevent post-herpetic neuralgia.

- Corticosteroids may be used in conjunction with antivirals, particularly if severe infection or lesions near the eyes are present.

- Amitryptyline, perphenazine, fluphenazine, or doxepin may be helpful in the treatment of post-herpetic neuralgia. Analgesics may also be necessary.

- Capsaicin ointment 0.025%, applied TID or QID is effective in the treatment of post-herpetic neuralgia in some individuals.

TRANSCULTURAL
NURSING

Transcultural Nursing

CULTURAL ASSESSMENT CONSIDERATIONS

Sensitivity to the client's culture is extremely important. Thorough cultural assessment is very time consuming. However, at a minimum, obtaining the following information will assist the nurse in planning care.

- Where was the client born? If the client is an immigrant, how long has he/she lived in the United States?

- What is the client's ethnic affiliation?

- Who are the client's significant others? Does the client reside in an ethnic community?

- What are the client's primary and secondary languages? Can the client speak and read in these languages?

- What is the client's nonverbal communication style?

- What is the client's religion and how important are religious practices in daily life?

- What are the client's food preferences? Food prohibitions?

- What is the client's current economic situation?

- Does the client have special health and illness beliefs and practices?

- Does the client have special beliefs surrounding transitional life events such as birth, illness, and death?

CULTURAL INTERPRETATION OF NONVERBAL COMMUNICATIONS AND PERSONAL SPACE

Culture	Nonverbal Communication
American (US)	Makes eye contact. Personal space 18" to 36"
American Indian	Avoiding eye contact is sign of respect. Distant personal space, not well defined.
Arab American	Women may avoid eye contact with males and non-acquaintances. Close personal space.
Brazilian	Lower class may avoid eye contact as a sign of respect. Close personal space.
Cambodian	Eye contact acceptable; women may lower eyes slightly. Close personal space.
Chinese American	Eye contact with authority figures avoided as a sign of respect; clients will make eye contact with family and friends. Distant personal space, not well defined.
Columbian	May not make eye contact in presence of an authority figure. Close personal space.
Cuban	Direct eye contact expected when speaking. Close personal space with friends and family.

Continued...

Culture	Nonverbal Communication
Ethiopian	Little eye contact with authority figures. Close personal space with family and friends.
Filipino	Little eye contact with authority figures. Close personal space.
Gypsy	Facial expressions often reflective of mood. Close personal space with family members; avoid close contact with non-Gypsies and surfaces considered unclean (areas where lower body has touched).
Haitian	Avoid eye contact with authority figures.
Hmong	Prolonged eye contact considered rude.
Iranian	Eye contact only between equals and close family and friends. Close personal space.
Japanese American	Little eye contact. Touching uncommon.
Korean	Little direct eye contact. Touching considered disrespectful. Close personal space with family; entering personal space is disrespectful.
Mexican American	Direct eye contact avoided with authority figures. Some perceive touch by strangers as disrespectful.

TRANSCULTURAL NURSING

Continued…

Culture	Nonverbal Communication
Puerto Rican	Personal space may vary with age; generally a reasonable distance in older women, closer with younger women.
Russian	Make direct eye contact during conversation. Close personal space with family and friends.
South Asian	Direct eye contact with elderly may be considered rude. Close personal space with family members.
Vietnamese	Eye contact with authority figures avoided. Distant personal space.
West Indian	Avoid eye contact. Distant personal space.

CULTURAL/RELIGIOUS BELIEFS AFFECTING CARE AT THE TIME OF DEATH

Culture/Religion	Religious Belief
Adventist (Seventh Day, Church of God)	Some groups believe in divine healing, anointing with oil, and prayer.
American Indian	Beliefs vary according to tribe. Some believe an owl is an omen of death. Family members prepare the body for burial in some tribes. Some tribes will not touch the dead person's belongings after death. Some believe the dead are happy in the spirit world. Others believe the body is an empty shell. Some have extensive preparation of the body and visitation of the deceased. If a member of some tribes dies at home, the house is abandoned forever, or may be burned.
Armenian Church	Holy Communion may be given as a form of last rites; practice laying on of hands
Baptist	Pastor, patient, and family counsel and pray. Some practice healing and laying on of hands.
Black/African American	Deceased is highly respected. Health care providers usually prepare the body. Cremation and organ donation are usually avoided.

Continued…

Culture/Religion	Religious Belief
Black Muslim	Practices for washing the body, applying the shroud, and funeral rites are carefully prescribed.
Brethren	Anointing with oil is done for physical healing and spiritual guidance.
Buddhist Churches of America	The priest is contacted. Chanting may be done at the bedside after death.
Cambodian (Khmer)	Family wants to be present at time of death and may want to care for the client. Incense may be burned. Monks recite prayers. Death is accepted in a quiet, passive manner. Family and monks may wish to prepare the body. A white cloth is used as a shroud and mourners wear white.
Central American	Catholics may want a priest to administer Sacrament of the Sick. Candles may be used if oxygen not in use in room. Family members may wish to prepare the body.
Chinese American	Family may prefer client not be told of impending death, or may prefer to inform the client themselves. May not want to talk about the terminal illness with anyone. Some believe that dying at home is bad luck. Others believe that

Continued...

Culture/Religion	Religious Belief
Chinese American (continued)	the spirit gets lost if the client dies in the hospital. Family members may place special cloths and amulets on the body. Some prefer to bathe family members after death.
Christian Scientist	A Christian Science Practitioner may be called for spiritual support.
Church of God	Believes in divine healing through prayer. May practice speaking in tongues.
Colombian	Catholic prayer and Anointing of the Sick common. Family may practice Catholic prayer at bedside. Family members may cry loudly or become hysterical. All family members may want to see the body before it is taken to the morgue. In Columbia, the deceased are usually buried within 24 to 36 hours. Family should be informed that in the US this may not happen as quickly.
Cuban	Family may not want client told of impending death. This varies according to Cuban culture. Family members may stay with client 24 hours a day during terminal phase of illness.

TRANSCULTURAL NURSING

Continued...

Culture/Religion	Religious Belief
Eastern Orthodox	Last rites are given. Anointing of the sick is performed as a form of healing with prayer.
Episcopal	Last rites are available, but not mandatory.
Ethiopian	Friends are told of death before family so they can be present for support when family is informed. Female family members are never told first. Very emotional at death and may cry loudly and hysterically. Women may tear their clothing and beat their chests. Men may cry out loud. Some families may want to say goodbye to the deceased before the body is removed from the room.
Filipino	Head of family is informed away from client's room. Catholic priest is called to deliver Sacrament of the Sick. Do not resuscitate decisions may be made by the entire family. Religious objects may be placed around the clientand family may pray at the bedside. After death, may cry loudly and hysterically. Family may wish to wash the body. Death is considered a very spiritual event. All family members may want to say goodbye before body is removed from the room.

Continued...

Culture/Religion	Religious Belief
Friends (Quaker)	Do not believe in life after death.
Greek Orthodox	The priest should be called while the client is still conscious. Practices last rites and administration of Holy Communion.
Gypsy	In general, discussion of death is avoided in this culture. Eldest in authority is informed of death first. A priest may be present for body purification. Family may want the window open at the time of death and afterward so the spirit can leave the room. May ask for special personal items in room at the time of death. An older female relative may remain at the window to keep spirits out of room. The moment of death and the client's last words are very significant. The body after death may represent a source of spiritual danger to the family. Family may want body embalmed immediately after death to remove blood. They may sit with the body around the clock after death, and will eat and drink in the room during this watch.

Continued...

TRANSCULTURAL NURSING

Culture/Religion	Religious Belief
Haitian	Elaborate rituals after death. Family will cry hysterically and uncontrollably when death imminent. Family members may bring religious symbols and medallions. They have a deep respect for the dead. Family members may wish to wash the body and participate in post-mortem care.
Hindu	Specially prescribed rites. Family members wash and dress the body and only certain persons may touch the dead.
Hmong	Client is dressed in fine traditional Hmong clothing at the time of death. Family may put amulets on body, which should not be removed. The family usually prepares the body at the funeral home. The body cannot be buried with hard objects, buttons, or zippers against the body.
Iranian	Death is seen as the beginning of a spiritual relationship with God, not end of life. Family may remain at the bedside at all times when client is dying, and may cry and pray. Families may wish to wash the body.

Continued...

Culture/Religion	Religious Belief
Islam (Muslim)	Begging forgiveness and confession of sins must be done in presence of family members before death. Five steps are used to prepare the body for burial. The body is washed by a Muslim of the same gender. May offer special prayers at bedside to ease pain and suffering. Some have spiritual leader give client holy water to drink prior to death to purify body. After death, arms and legs are straightened and the toes tied together with a bandage.
Japanese	Client and family may be aware of impending death, but will not speak about it. Family may wish to remain at bedside during terminal stage of illness. Cleanliness and dignity of the body are important.
Judaism (Orthodox and Conservative)	Church members wash and prepare the body.
Korean	Chanting, incense, and praying may be used. Family may be very emotional. Family may want to spend time alone with client after death. Some may wish to wash the body.

TRANSCULTURAL NURSING

Continued…

Culture/Religion	Religious Belief
Lutheran	Last rites optional; the client may request anointing of the sick.
Mexican American	Entire family may be obligated to visit the sick and dying. Pregnant women may be prohibited from visiting. Spiritual items may be important. May want to die at home because of the fear that the spirit will get lost in the hospital. Crying loudly and wailing is culturally accepted and a sign of respect. A Catholic priest is called for the Sacrament of the Sick. A family member may wish to assist with post-mortem care. Family will want time alone with the body before it is removed from the room.
Orthodox Presbyterian	Scripture reading and prayer.
Puerto Rican	Family may stay around the clock if death is imminent. Some believe that all immediate family members must be present at time of death. Puerto Ricans believe the body must be treated with great respect.

Continued…

Culture/Religion	Religious Belief
Roman Catholic	The Rite for Anointing of the Sick is desired. Client or family may request anointing if prognosis is poor.
Russian	Family may not want client to know of terminal diagnosis. Depending on religion, family may wish to wash the body and dress it in special clothes.
Russian Orthodox	Many wear a cross necklace, which should not be removed, if at all possible. After death the arms are crossed, and fingers set in the form of a cross. Clothing must be a natural fiber so the body changes to ashes sooner.
Samoan	Client and family prefer to be told of terminal diagnosis as early as possible. Family would prefer to care for client at home. Family members usually prepare the body.
Sikh	Believe that the soul remains alive after death. Family washes the body and dresses in new clothes.
Vietnamese	DNR decisions are made by entire family. For Catholic families, religious items are kept close to client. For Buddhist families, incense is burned. Families prefer time alone with the deceased before body is removed. The

TRANSCULTURAL NURSING

Continued...

Culture/Religion	Religious Belief
Vietnamese (continued)	body is highly respected, and the family may prefer to wash it. Some may prefer the body left as it is.
West Indian	When death is near, close family and friends remain at the bedside for prayer. Family members may wish to view the body exactly as the client was at the time of death. Most wish to be alone with the deceased.

Nursing

Considerations

Nursing Considerations

CLIENT AND FAMILY EDUCATION

The Joint Commission takes the patient and family education (PF) standards very seriously. Client teaching deficiencies have been among the top 15 findings in health care facility surveys for several years.

PF.2.1 says clients and/or, when appropriate, their families must have their learning needs, abilities, learning preferences, and readiness to learn assessed.

PF.2.1.1 says education assessments should, when indicated, include cultural and religious practices, emotional barriers, desire and motivation to learn, physical and/or cognitive limitations, language barriers, and the financial implications of care choices.

PF.2.2.3 says hospitals should instruct clients and/or family on food/drug interactions as well as nutrition interventions and modified diets.

Recommendations:

- Document all client teaching.

- Avoid depending on the care plan as the only evidence of client teaching.

- Avoid long, technical instructions that clients cannot understand.

- Translate client teaching instructions into languages used by community populations.

- Assess the affect of cultural and religious practices on client teaching.

- Health care agencies should have clear policies outlining accountability and responsibilities for who does what.

- Develop a good, comprehensive assessment form that includes answers to the following questions:
  - How does this client learn best?
  - Is this client ready to learn?
  - Is the teaching material understandable?
  - What did I teach the client?
  - How do I know the client learned?

- Orient all relevant staff on the facility policies and the assessment form.

- Conduct a concurrent chart review to see if policies are implemented and being used.

THE PATIENT SELF DETERMINATION ACT

The Patient Self Determination Act (PSDA) became effective in 1991. The purpose of the law is to ensure that clients are given information about their rights to execute an advance directive.

The PSDA requires hospitals, nursing facilities, and other health care providers who receive federal

Medicare or Medicaid funds to offer clients written information explaining their legal options for accepting or refusing treatment in the event they are incapacitated.

The PSDA laws vary from state to state. The significant provisions of the act are:

1. Hospitals, nursing facilities, home health care agencies, hospice, and HMO's are required to maintain written policies and procedures guaranteeing clients written information explaining their involvement in treatment decisions. The information provided must provide state-specific information, and written policies of the health care organization regarding implementation of these rights. The medical record must contain documentation regarding whether the client has implemented an advanced directive.

2. The health care agency must provide for education of staff and the community regarding advance directives.

3. Each state is required to develop written descriptions of the law concerning advance directives in their jurisdiction, and provide this material to health care providers.

Nurses' Responsibility

The American Nurses Association published a statement describing the nurses' responsibilities in implementation of the PSDA. The ANA recommendations state that nurses should be familiar with the laws of the state in which they practice, and should be familiar with the strengths and limitations of each form of advance directive. They further state that the nurse has the responsibility to facilitate informed decision making, including, but not limited to advance directives.

The Legal Documents

All states have laws providing for designation of a durable power of attorney, developing a living will, or both. Each state has specific laws regarding who may witness the execution of these documents. The nurse must be aware of specific laws for the state in which he or she practices.

- **Living Wills** state the client's wishes regarding medical treatment in the event of a terminal illness or condition.

- **The Durable Power of Attorney for Health Care** designates another person to make health care decisions for the client if he or she loses the ability to make decisions. The role of the designated individual in this situation is to make decisions that most closely align with the values, wishes, and desires of the client.

ELDER ABUSE

The elderly are not immune from the increasing violence in society today. It is estimated that abuse, neglect, and mistreatment of the elderly occurs in 4% to 10% of the aged population. Each state defines abuse in a slightly different manner. Nurses are mandatory reporters of suspected abuse in many states. Abuse can occur in the community as well as institutional settings.

Types of Abuse

Physical abuse	Physical contact that causes physical pain or mental distress. Physical abuse includes hitting, slapping, burning, pushing, or leaving the client in unsafe physical conditions.
Neglect	Deliberately not caring for the client. Examples of neglect include unexplained weight loss, pressure ulcers, dehydration, and contractures.
Sexual Abuse	Any form of unwelcome sexual contact by force or threat of

	force. Indications of sexual abuse include difficulty walking, sitting, or urinating, bruising or bleeding of the external genitalia, and the presence of blood in undergarments.
Emotional Abuse	Making threats of violence, removal, or withdrawal of care and services.
Financial Exploitation	Taking advantage of the elderly for financial or material gain.
Abandonment	Willfully deserting the client or withdrawing care.
Mistreatment	Administering medications or treatments to control the elderly client. For example, restraining a client to a chair when restraints are not necessary, or administering a psychotropic drug to control behavior when no problem exists.
Self Abuse or Neglect	The elderly client is unable to meet his or her own activities of daily living or instrumental activities of daily living, but refuses the help of others.

Signs and Symptoms of Abuse and Neglect

Signs and symptoms of abuse vary widely. By themselves, these factors do not necessarily mean an abusive situation exists. If one or more of the following are present, they may be indications of abuse or neglect.

- Client is dirty or dressed inappropriately
- Unkempt appearance
- Client appears malnourished, but has a good appetite.
- Reluctance of the client to discuss the problem.
- Prolonged period between the illness or injury and request for care.
- The severity of an injury does not correspond with the explanation of events.
- Client may make disparaging remarks about family members
- Client may appear passive, elusive, or frightened.
- Client appears overmedicated.
- Depression
- Infantile behavior
- Withdrawal, unwilling to talk
- Agitation
- Injuries in various stages of healing

- Has pressure sores that have not been cared for adequately.
- Unexplained bruising, lacerations, or skin tears
- Pain, itching, bruising, or bleeding in the genital area.
- Stained, torn, or bloody undergarments.
- Broken teeth
- Eye injuries
- Fractures, particularly transverse or oblique fractures of long bones

The caregiver:

- Does not want the health care professional to be alone with the client.
- May appear hostile and angry
- Pressures client into signing legal documents or checks
- Complains excessively about caring for the client
- Does not provide medication or proper care
- Does not keep the client clean or appropriately dressed

NURSING

CARE PLANNING

Nursing Care Planning

THE NURSING PROCESS

The nursing process is a systematic process consisting of five steps:

1. Assessment of the client's health data
2. Analysis of data and formulation of a nursing diagnosis
3. Planning priorities for client care
4. Implementation of the plan according to priorities and planned outcome criteria
5. Evaluation of the client's response and revision of the plan as necessary

Assessment consists of an initial and ongoing process of the client's status. Upon completion of the assessment, the nurse makes a complete diagnostic statement to guide the care plan. Nursing diagnoses are listed according to priority and are based on a mutual client-nurse decision. Realistic care plan priorities are developed to meet the client's individual needs. The plan is implemented, with the nurse constantly assessing the effectiveness and ineffectiveness of the approaches. The client's progress is evaluated based on designated outcome criteria. The plan is continually reassessed, modified, and updated to assist the client to achieve the established goals.

NURSING INTERVENTIONS CLASSIFICATION

The Nursing Interventions Classification (NIC) was developed by a team of nurse researchers at the University of Iowa. It was first published in 1992, and subsequently revised in 1996. The system is linked to NANDA diagnosis, and is being adopted by multiple clinical and educational agencies.

A nursing intervention is defined as *any treatment, based upon clinical judgment and knowledge, that a nurse performs to enhance patient/client outcomes.*[1] Nursing interventions include both direct and indirect care and may be initiated by the nurse, physician, or other health care provider. Interventions may include both direct and indirect care. NIC is a standardized listing of nursing interventions that can be used in all practice settings to assist in the resolution of the client's real and potential problems. Implementing the classification system will do much to advance nursing practice as we approach the 21st century.

Prior to selecting nursing interventions, the nurse specifies desired client outcomes. The effectiveness of the intervention is measured by the outcome. Outcomes and interventions are designed to alter the causative factors associated with the diagnosis and are selected in relation to the NANDA diagnosis. The client's status will improve if the causative factors are eliminated or altered. If the causative factors cannot be altered, the intervention will be selected to treat signs and symptoms. Some nursing diagnoses are designated as "risk." When an intervention is selected for a risk

nursing diagnosis, the intevention will alter or eliminate risk factors.

The Nursing Interventions Classifications currently
consists of 433 interventions. Each intervention
consists of a label name, definition, and list of
activities to carry out the intervention. A listing of
background readings is included with each
intervention to provide the nurse with resources for
further information. Each intervention provides
research-based practice activities from which to
develop and revise the care plan. Nursing interventions
define treatments that nurses perform and that
enhance communication among health care providers.
Use of nursing interventions promotes advancement of
nursing clinical knowledge and provides nurses with an
opportunity to gain a greater voice in the health care
policy arena. The client will realize many tangible
benefits from the use of this system.

NURSING OUTCOMES CLASSIFICATION

The Nursing Outcomes Classification (NOC) is
linked to NANDA nursing diagnoses. As of 1977, there
are 190 nursing outcomes with indicators for nurses to
evaluate the effectiveness of interventions. Client
progress is easily measured by using the nursing outcomes. Each nursing outcome consists of a label name,
definition, set of indicators, and measurement scale.
Like the Nursing Interventions Classification, the outcomes classification provides selected references for
additional research and information.

Measuring client progress and outcomes has long been a problem for the nursing profession. The Nursing Outcomes Classification provides nurses with a tool to measure the client's progress or regression on a daily basis, and revise the plan of care accordingly. Nursing outcomes are also used at the time of discharge. If the client has not made optimal progress, referral can be made to the appropriate agency.

Current trends in health care delivery stress consumer satisfaction and outcome evaluation as criteria for selecting health care providers. Census is the key to maintaining health care facility operations and preserving jobs for health care providers. Consumers have many agencies to chose from. Attention to customer satisfaction has become a key to survival in the health care industry. Facilities across the nation are downsizing and restructuring. *"As the nursing profession struggles to retain its identity in a health care system being restructured for greater efficiency, the need for nursing to define its interventions and outcomes has never been greater."*[2]

The use of nursing diagnoses, standardized language for nursing interventions and nursing outcomes provides a logical, organized system for the gerontological nurse to use to maximize the effectiveness of the nursing process.

---

[1] Nursing Interventions Classification (NIC), 2/E, Joanne McCloskey, Gloria Bulechek, © 1996 Mosby-Year Book, Inc.

[2] Nursing Outcomes Classification (NOC), Marion Johnson, Meridean Maas, © Mosby-Year Book, Inc. 1997

NANDA Approved Nursing Diagnoses

Activity Intolerance

Activity Intolerance, Risk for

Adaptive capacity: Intracranial, Decreased

Adjustment, Impaired

Airway Clearance, Ineffective

Anxiety

Aspiration, Risk for

Body Image Disturbance

Body Temperature, Risk for Altered

Breastfeeding, Effective

Breastfeeding, Ineffective

Breastfeeding, Interrupted

Breathing Pattern, Ineffective

Cardiac Output, Decreased

Caregiver Role Strain

Caregiver Role Strain, Risk for

Communication, Impaired Verbal

Community Coping, Ineffective

Community Coping, Potential for Enhanced

Confusion, Acute

Confusion, Chronic

Constipation

Constipation, Colonic

Constipation, Perceived

Coping, Defensive

Coping, Ineffective Individual

Decisional Conflict (Specify)

Denial, Ineffective

Diarrhea

Disuse Syndrome, Risk for

Diversional Activity Deficit

Dysfunctional Ventilatory Weaning Response

Dysreflexia

Energy Field, Disturbance

Environmental Interpretation Syndrome, Impaired

Family Coping: Compromised, Ineffective

Family Coping: Disabling, Ineffective

Family Coping: Potential for Growth

Family Processes, Altered

Family Processes, Altered: Alcoholism

Fatigue

Fear

Fluid Volume Deficit

Fluid Volume Deficit, Risk for

Fluid Volume Excess

Gas Exchange, Impaired

Grieving, Anticipatory

Grieving, Dysfunctional

Growth and Development, Altered

Health Maintenance, Altered

Health-Seeking Behaviors (Specify)

Home Maintenance Management, Impaired

Hopelessness

Hyperthermia

Hypothermia

Incontinence, Bowel

Incontinence, Functional

Incontinence, Reflex

Incontinence, Stress

Incontinence, Total

Incontinence, Urge

Infant Behavior, Disorganized

Infant Behavior, Risk for Disorganized

Infant Behavior, Potential for Enhanced Organized

Infant Feeding Pattern, Ineffective

Infection, Risk for

Injury, Risk for

Knowledge Deficit (specify)

Loneliness, Risk for

Management of Therapeutic Regimen, Effective

Management of Therapeutic Regimen:Community, Ineffective

Management of Therapeutic Regimen: Families, Ineffective

Management of Therapeutic Regimen: Individual, Effective

Management of Therapeutic Regimen: Individual, Ineffective

Memory, Impaired

Noncompliance (Specify)

Nutrition: Less than Body Requirements, Altered

Nutrition: More than Body Requirements, Altered

Nutrition: Risk for More than Body Requirements, Altered

Oral Mucous Membrane, Altered

Pain

Pain, Chronic

Parent / Infant / Child Attachment, Risk for Altered

Parental Role Conflict

Parenting, Altered

Parenting, Risk for Altered

Perioperative Positioning; Risk for Injury

Peripheral Neurovascular Dysfunction, Risk for

Personal Identity Disturbance

Physical Mobility, Impaired

Poisoning, Risk for

Post-Trauma Response

Powerlessness

Protection, Altered

Rape-Trauma Syndrome

Rape-Trauma Syndrome: Compound Reaction

Rape-Trauma Syndrome: Silent Reaction

Relocation Stress Syndrome

Role Performance, Altered

Self-Care Deficit: Feeding, Bathing/Hygiene,
Dressing/Grooming, Toileting

Self Esteem, Chronic Low

Self Esteem, Situational Low

Self Esteem, Disturbance

Self-Mutilation, Risk for

Sensory/Perceptual Alteration (Specify Type: Visual,
Auditory, Kinesthetic, Gustatory, Tactile, and Olfactory)

Sexual Dysfunction

Sexuality Patterns, Altered

Skin Integrity, Impaired

Skin Integrity, Risk for Impaired

Sleep Pattern Disturbance

Social Interaction, Impaired

Social Isolation

Spiritual Distress (Distress of the Human Spirit)

Spiritual Well-Being, Potential for Enhanced

Suffocation, Risk for

Swallowing, Impaired

Thermoregulation, Ineffective

Thought Processes, Altered

Tissue Integrity, Impaired

Tissue Perfusion, Altered Cardiac

Tissue Perfusion, Altered (Specify Type: Renal, Cerebral, Cardiopulmonary, Gastrointestinal, Peripheral)

Trauma, Risk for

Unilateral Neglect

Urinary Elimination, Altered

Urinary Retention

Ventilation, Inability to Sustain Spontaneous

Violence, Risk for: Self-directed or Directed at Others

FINANCING

HEALTH CARE

FINANCING HEALTH CARE

MEDICARE COVERAGE

Medicare is a health insurance programs for individuals age 65 or over. Disabled individuals under age 65 qualify for Medicare coverage after 24 months of disability. Individuals with end stage renal disease and dialysis are eligible for coverage without the 24 month waiting period.

The provider of the service must be Medicare approved.

The two components to the Medicare program are:

Part A-Hospital Insurance

Pays for medically necessary in-patient hospital and skilled nursing facility care.

Part B-Medical Insurance

Participation in Part B is optional. This service can be purchased by individuals who do not qualify for Part A. If coverage is accepted by the individual, there is a monthly charge, which is deducted from the Social Security check. Part B pays for medically necessary physician and outpatient services. For services covered under Part B, Medicare pays 80% of the cost of service and the client pays 20%.

In-Patient services covered under Part A in the hospital:

Hospital room and board

Nursing and related services

Operating and recovery room costs

Diagnostic and therapeutic services

In Patient services covered under Part A in the skilled nursing facility:

Semi-private room and ancillaries

Drugs (while under Part A)

Medical supplies (while under Part A)

Physical, occupational, speech, and respiratory therapy (while under Part A)

Laboratory services (while under Part A)

X-Ray (while under Part A)

Oxygen (while under Part A)

Medicare imposes significant restrictions on payment for care in long-term care facilities. The client's condition is the determining factor regarding whether he or she qualifies for coverage. The client must require a daily skilled nursing or rehabilitation service that can only be provided by, or under the supervision of, licensed health care personnel. Coverage ceases when the client no longer requires a daily skilled service. Very few individuals qualify for the full 100 day benefit period in a long-term care facility.

Long-term care facility benefits operate on a "spell of illness" concept. The client may qualify for repeated 100 day benefit periods if the spell of illness is broken. To "break" the spell of illness, the client must not require a daily skilled service for 60 consecutive days or must go home for 60 consecutive days. Prior to admission to the Medicare program in a skilled nursing facility, the client must spend three consecutive nights (four days) in an acute care hospital.

Services covered under Medicare Part B

Physician services and supplies
Hospital outpatient services
Diagnostic lab and x-ray
X-Ray therapy
Surgical dressings and supplies
Ambulance
Durable medical equipment
Prosthetic devices
Braces, trusses, artificial limbs
Catheters and supplies
Tube feeding solutions and supplies
Colostomy bags and supplies
Outpatient therapy services
Pneumococcal, influenza, and Hepatitis B vaccine
Portable dialysis systems
Outpatient dialysis

MEDICAID COVERAGE

Medicaid is a combined state and federal program. Each governmental entity contributes a portion of the cost of health care.

Medicaid provides medical assistance for low income individuals of all ages who cannot pay for medical care, providing they meet income requirements. The state agency that administers the program determines who is eligible within certain federal limits and income/asset eligibility guidelines. The benefits differ in each state.

The Medicaid program is state-administered and pays a set rate according to the state Medicaid program allowables. It may or may not cover all medical expenses. Some services and drugs require prior authorization.

LONG-TERM CARE HEALTH INSURANCE

There are two basic types of long-term care insurance: home health care and nursing home care. Medicare supplement policies are sold by private insurance companies and fill some of the gaps in Medicare coverage. Hospital deductibles and excess physicians' charges are routinely covered, but many policies do not cover long-term care expenses.

Long-term care insurance policies must be cautiously evaluated. Many policies contain loopholes that do not adequately protect a senior's life savings. Some policies have such strict disability criteria that many policyholders do not qualify for benefits. One of the keys to evaluating long-term care insurance is to read the policy itself. Disregard promotional literature, which can be misleading.

Insurers carefully limit and control where the client can receive services. Unless the client receives services in an approved facility, the insurer will refuse to pay for care. Many insurers will not cover custodial care. Some will describe the types of facilities where clients will not be covered.

Insurance policies are many and varied and most have restrictions on the type of services provided. Common descriptions include the type of nursing supervision, the size of the facility, type of care provided, and level of licensing. Many will not pay for long-term care unless the client qualifies for long-term care services under the Medicare program. Policies that require the beneficiary to receive only "skilled" care are virtually worthless. Most long-term care facility residents do not require skilled care according to the accepted definition. Some insurers do not use the Medicare qualifying requirements, but do require the facility to be Medicare certified.

The best long-term care policies pay for services ordered by the physician. However, some insurers require that care be "medically necessary for sickness and injury." The insurance company makes the determination whether the services are medically necessary, not the attending physician. Some policies provide benefits if clients require assistance with ADL's. However, the definitions used to describe activities of daily living varies with the insurer, so reading the policy definitions is important. Like Medicare, some insurers require the three night hospital stay. A governmental study shows that 57% of all individuals entering a long-term care facility do not have an acute illness requiring prior hospitalization. Some policies pay for services related only to acute illness. Note the definition of "acute" carefully. If the client has an underlying chronic condition, it may be difficult to differentiate the reason long-term care services are required.

Many policies are "service based." This means that the client must require specific services in order to qualify for coverage. Regardless of the type or level of disability, clients are limited to receiving particularly defined services at specific facilities.

Several private companies can provide information on how analysts view particular insurance companies. Ratings are available at most public libraries, or the agencies listed below can be contacted directly:

Best Company (900) 420-0400

Demotech, Inc. (614) 761-8602

Duff & Phelps, Inc. (312) 368-3157

Fitch Investors Service, Inc. (212) 908-0500

Moody's Investor Service (212) 553-1653

Standard & Poor's (212) 208-1527

Weiss Research, Inc. (800) 289-9222

The United States General Accounting Office published a special report to the U.S. House of Representatives, entitled Insurance Ratings: Comparison of Private Agency Ratings for Life/Health Insurers [GAO/GGD-94-2094BR]. The report may be purchased for $2 by writing U.S. General Accounting Office, P.O. Box 6015, Gaithersburg, MD 20884-6015.

CLINICAL

REFERRALS

CLINICAL REFERRALS

RESOURCES FOR GERONTOLOGICAL NURSES

Alliance for Aging Research
2021 K St. NW, Suite 305
Washington, DC 20006
(202) 293-2856
(202) 785-8574-fax

American Association for Homes and Services for the
Aging
901 E Street NW, Suite 500
Washington, DC 20004-2037
(202) 508-9472
(202) 783-2255-fax

American Association of Retired Persons
1909 K Street NW
Washington, D.C. 20049
(202) 434-2277

American College of Health Care Administrators
325 S. Patrick St.
Alexandria, VA 22314
(703) 739-7900
(703) 739-7901-fax

American Geriatrics Society
770 Lexington Avenue, Suite 300
New York, NY 10021
(212) 308-1414
(212) 832-8646-fax
http://www.wwilkins.com/AGS

American Health Care Association
1201 L Street, NW
Washington, DC 20005
(202) 842-4444
(202) 842-3860-fax

American Medical Directors Association
(Long-Term Care)
10480 Little Patuxent Parkway, Suite 760
Columbia, MD 21044
(800) 876-AMDA
(410) 740-9743
(410) 740-4572-fax

American Nurses Association, Inc.
Council on Gerontological Nursing
2420 Pershing Road
Kansas City, MO 64108

American Public Health Association Section on
Gerontological Health
1015 18th Street, NW
Washington, D.C. 20036

American Society for Long-Term Care Nurses
660 Lonely Cottage Drive
Upper Black Eddy, PA 18972
(610) 847-5396
(610) 847-5063-fax

American Society of Consultant Pharmacists
1321 Duke St.
Alexandria, VA 22314-3563
(703) 739-1300
(703) 739-1321-fax

American Society on Aging
833 Market Street, Suite 512
San Francisco, CA 94103
(415) 543-2617

Assisted Living Facilities Association of America
10300 Eaton Place, Suite 400
Farfax, VA 22030
(703) 691-8100
(703) 691-8106-fax

Association for Gerontology in Higher Education
600 Maryland Avenue SW
West Wing 204
Washington, D.C. 20024
(202) 484-7505

Gerontological Society of America
1275 K Street, NW, Suite 350
Washington, DC 20006
(202) 842-1275
(202) 842-1150-fax

Hospice Association of America
228 7th Street, SE
Washington, DC 20003
(202) 546-4759

National Association for Home Care
205 C Street, NE
Washington, D.C. 20002

National Association of Adult Day Care
180 East 4050 South
Murray, UT 84107
(801) 262-9167

National Association of Area Agencies on Aging
1112 16th Street NW, Suite 100
Washington, D.C . 20036
(202) 296-8130

National Association of Directors of Nursing
Administration in Long-Term Care
10999 Reed Hartman Highway
Suite 229
Cincinnati, OH 45242-8301
(800) 222-0539
(513) 791-3699-fax

National Association of Home Health Agencies
426 C Street NE, Suite 200
Washington, D.C. 20002
(202) 547-1717

National Association of Private Geriatric Care
Managers
1604 North Country Club Road
Tucson, AZ 85716
(602) 881-8008

National Citizens Coalition for Nursing Home
Reform
1424 16th Street NW, Suite L-2
Washington, DC 20036
(202) 332-2275

National Council on the Aging, Inc.
409 Third Street, SW, Suite 202
Washington, D.C. 20024

National Council on Senior Citizens
925 15th Street NW
Washington, DC 20036
(202) 479-1200

National Family Caregivers Association
9621 E. Bexhill Drive
Kensington, MO 20895-3104
(800) 896-3650
e-mail CAREGIVING@aol.com

National Gerontological Nursing Association
11401 Georgia Avenue, Suite 203
Wheaton, MD 20902

National Home Caring Council
235 Park Avenue South
New York, NY 10003

National Institute on Adult Day Care
600 Maryland Ave SW
Washington, D.C. 20024
(202) 479-1200

National League of Nursing
Council of Community Health Services
10 Columbus Circle
New York, NY 10019
(212) 582-1022

National Subacute Care Association
7315 Wisconsin Avenue, Suite 424E
Bethesda, MD 20814
(301) 961-8680
(301) 961-8681-fax

INTERNET RESOURCES

The following is a listing of internet resources related to gerontological nursing. Many of these resources are linked to other sites, providing a comprehensive data base for gerontological nursing information.

1-800 Numbers for Patient Support
    http://infonet.welch.jhu.edu/advocacy.html

Academic Journal Directory
    http://www.son.utmb.edu/catalog/catalog.htm

Administration on Aging
    http://www.aoa.dhhs.gov

AOA Resources and links
    http://www.aoa.dhhs.gov/aoa/pages/jpostlst.html

Advanced Directives International
    http://www.adiwills.com/index.html

American Association of Retired Persons
    http://www.aarp.org

Directory of Web Aging Sites
    http://www.aoa.dhhs.gov/aoa/webres/craig.htm

Duke University Center for the Study of Aging and

Human Development
http://www.geri.duke.edu/ltc/ltc2.html

Eldercare Resource Locator
http://www.aoa.dhhs.gov/aoa/pages/loctrnew.html

Geriatric Data Bases
http://gsa.iog.wayne.edu/data.html

Gerisource
http://www.gerisource.com

Gerontological Nursing Resources on the
World Wide Web
http://www.uncg.edu/nur/gerohome.htm
http://www.uncg.edu:80/nur/gerohome.htm

Gerontological Library
http://www.usc.edu/Library/gero/

The GeroWeb Virtual Library on Aging
http://geriatricspt.org/othersites/internet.html

Global Community Nursing Site
   http://www.utexas.edu/nursing/fac-staff-
   stu/pages/glob-com-nurs/glob-com-nurs.html

Hardin Meta Directory-Geriatrics
   http://www.arcade.uiowa.edu/hardin-www/md-
   ger.html

Healthweb-Geriatrics and Gerontology
   http://www.uic.edu/depts/lib/health/hw/ger

HELP Magazine for long-term Care Nurses
   http://PSLN1.psln.com/helpPubs

Huffington Center on Aging
   http://www.bcm.tmc.edu/hcoa

Internet Infection Control Resources for long-term
Care Facilities
   http://BroadStreetSolutions.com

Long-term Care Today
   http://www.longtermcaretoday.com

Minimum Data Set 2.0 Web Sites
   http://linear.chsra.wisc.edu/mds_info.htm
   http://www.hcfa.gov/medicare/hsqb/mds20

Mr. long-term Care
   http://www.Mr-longtermcare.com

Martindale's Virtual Nursing Center
   http://www.sci.lib.uci.edu/~martindale/nursing.html

National Institute on Aging
   http://www.senior.com/npo/nia.html

National Aging Information Center
   http://www.ageinfo.org

National Gerontological Nursing Association
   http://www.ajn.org/ajnnet/nrsorgs/ngna

Nursing Interventions Classification, University of
Iowa
   http://www.nursing.uiowa.edu/nic

Nursing Outcomes Classification, University of Iowa
    http://www.nursing.uiowa.edu/noc

Nursing Home and long-term Care Topics
    http://www.geocities.com/HotSprings/2021

Nursing Resources
    http://www.access.digex.net/~nurse/website.htm

Nursing Societies and Organizations
    http://www.gen.emory.edu/MEDWEB/keyword/societies_and_associations.html

Online Resources for Geriatric Nurses
    http://www.geriatricvideo.com/resource.htm

Springhouse Books (links to sites of interest for
nurses and managers)
    http://www.springnet.com

UTMB Center on Aging
    http://www.utmb.edu/aging/index.html

Government Agencies

Master Listing of Government Agencies
http://metro.turnpike.net/adorn/gov.html

Agency for Toxic Substances and Disease Registry
http://atsdr1.cdc.gov:8080/atsdrhome.html

Agency for Health Care Policy and Research
(AHCPR) Guidelines
http://www.ahcpr.gov

Centers for Disease Control
http://www.cdc.gov

CDC Wonder Data Base
http://wonder.cdc.gov

Food and Drug Administration (FDA)
http://www.fda.gov

Government Publications Office
http://www.gpo.ucop.edu

Health Care Financing Administration (HCFA)
    http://www.hcfa.gov

Department of Health and Human Services
    http://www.os.dhhs.gov

Health and Human Services Agencies
    http://www.os.dhhs.gov/progorg/progorg.html

Medline Data Base
    http://www.nlm.nih.gov

Morbidity and Mortality Weekly Report (MMWR)
    http://www.cdc.gov/epo/mmwr/mmwr.html

National Institutes of Health (NIH)
    http://www.nih.gov

National Library of Medicine
    http://www.nnlm.nlm.nih.gov/index.html

Occupational Safety and Health Administration (OSHA)

http://www.osha.gov

Social Security Administration

http://www.ssa.gov

U.S. Public Health Service

http://phs.os.dhhs.gov/phs/phs.html

ORGANIZATIONS FOR SPECIFIC PROBLEMS/CONDITIONS

The following is a list of telephone numbers of organizations devoted to client education for specific problems, conditions, and diseases.

Abuse

800-422-4453 National Child Abuse Hotline

800-222-2000 National Council on Child Abuse and Family Violence

Advocacy

201-625-7101 American Self-Help Clearinghouse

800-48-FRIEND The Friends' Health Connection

407-253-9048 Med Help International

Aging

800-424-3410 American Association of Retired Persons

202-434-2200 National Eldercare Institute on Health Promotion

800-222-3937 National Eye Care Project

800-222-2225 National Institute on Aging Information

AIDS

800-458-5231 National AIDS Information Clearinghouse

800-342-AIDS National AIDS Hotline

800-669-0696 AIDS Education at Work

800-673-8538 National Association of People with AIDS

Alcohol

800-622-2255 National Council on Alcoholism and Drug Dependancy

800-344-2666 Al-Anon, Alateen Family Group Hotline

800-527-5344 American Council on Alcoholism

800-729-6686 National Clearinghouse for Alcohol and Drug Information

800-354-7089 Alcohol Rehab for the Elderly

Allergy

800-822-2762 American Academy of Allergy Asthma & Immunology

800-727-8462 Asthma and Allergy Foundation of America

Alzheimer's

800-272-3900 Alzheimer's Association

800-477-2243 French Foundation for Alzheimer's Research

Americans with Disabilities Act

800-669-4000 Equal Employment Opportunity Commission (EEOC)

Amyotrophic Lateral Sclerosis

800-782-4747 Amyotrophic Lateral Sclerosis Association

Anorexia/Bulimia

847-831-3438 National Association of Anorexia Nervosa & Associated Disorders

Arthritis

800-283-7800 Arthritis Foundation

800-327-3027 Arthritis Consulting Services

614-881-5601 The Road Back Foundation

Asthma

800-822-2762 American Academy of Allergy Asthma & Immunology

800-LUNG-USA American Lung Association

800-727-8462 Asthma and Allergy Foundation of America

Ataxia

800-5-HELP-AT Ataxia Telangiectasia Childrens Project

612-473-7666 National Ataxia Foundation

Back Pain

800-247-2225 Back Pain Hotline

Biliary Atresia

718-987-6200 Biliary Atresia and Liver Transplant Network

Birth Defects

800-221-6827 National Easter Seal Society

Blind/Vision Impaired

800-683-5555 Foundation Fighting Blindness

800-424-8666 American Council of the Blind

800-232-5463 American Foundation for the Blind

800-562-6265 National Association of Parents of Visually Impaired

800-334-5497 National Center for Vision and Aging

800-548-4337 Guide Dog Foundation for the Blind

800-424-8567 National Library Services for the Blind and Physically Handicapped

Brain Aneurysms
617-723-3870 Brain Aneurysm Foundation

Brain Tumors
800-886-2282 American Brain Tumor Association
800-934-CURE National Brain Tumor Foundation

Burn Injuries
800-888-BURN The Phoenix Society

Cancer
510-204-4286 Alta Bates-Herrick Breast Cancer Risk Counseling
800-525-3777 AMC Information and Counseling Line
800-ACS-2345 American Cancer Society
800-LUNG-USA American Lung Association

412-422-BCIS Breast Cancer Information Service

800-4-CANCER Cancer Information Service

800-843-8114 American Institute for Cancer Research

301-984-9496 The Association of Community Cancer Centers

800-813-HOPE Cancer Care

800-366-2223 Candelighters Childhood Cancer Foundation

800-55-CHEMO CHEMOcare

800-ICARE-61 The International Cancer Alliance, Inc.

800-452-CURE International Myeloma Foundation

212-719-0154 National Alliance of Breast Cancer Organizations (NABCO)

202-296-7477 National Breast Cancer Coalition

800-4-CANCER National Cancer Institute

301-650-8868 National Coalition for Cancer Survivorship

301-496-7403 NCI's CancerFax

616-453-1477 Patient Advocates for Advanced Cancer Treatment

212-719-0364 SHARE

800-IM-AWARE The Susan G. Komen Breast Cancer Foundation

800-808-7866 US TOO International (Prostate Cancer/BPH)

800-221-2141 Y-ME Breast Cancer Organization (24 hrs: 312-986-8228)

Cerebral Palsy

800-872-5827 United Cerebral Palsy Association, Inc.

Children

800-433-9016 American Academy of Pediatrics

800-422-4453 Child Help USA

800-787-KIDS Children's Rights Council

800-872-5437 Missing Children Help Center

800-843-5678 National Center for Missing and Exploited Children

800-422-4453 National Child Abuse Hotline

800-892-5437 Kidsrights

800-222-2000 National Council on Child Abuse and Family Violence

Cleft Palate

800-242-5338 National Cleft Palate Association

Cocaine

800-262-2463 National Cocaine Hotline

800-347-8998 Cocaine Anonymous

Colitis

800-343-3637 National Foundation for Colitis and Ileitis

Consumer Health Information

800-821-6671 Consumer Health Information Research Institute

Consumer Product Safety

800-638-2772 Consumer Product Safety Commission

Crohn's/Colitis

800-343-3637 Crohn's and Colitis Foundation of America

Chronic Fatigue Syndrome

800-442-3437 CFIDS

Cultural Issues
888-432-5470 Transcultural Nursing Society

Cystic Fibrosis
800-344-4823 Cystic Fibrosis Foundation

Deafness
800-535-3323 Deafness Research Foundation

Depression
800-826-3632 National Depressive & Manic-Depressive Association
800-248-4344 National Foundation for Depressive Illness
410-955-4647 Depression and Related Affective Disorders Association
516-829-0091 National Alliance for Research on Schizophrenia and Depression
212-533-6374 Mood Disorders Support Group/NY
800-789-CMHS National Mental Health Services Knowledge Exchange Network

Diabetes

800-338-DMED American Association of Diabetes Educators

800-223-1138 Juvenile Diabetes Foundation

800-232-3472 American Diabetes Foundation

Disabilities

407-880-9232 American Association of Disabled Persons

800-962-9629 National Spinal Cord Injury Association

800-526-3456 National Spinal Cord Injury Hotline

800-248-2253 National Organization on Disability

800-346-2742 National Rehabilitation Information Center

800-922-9234 National Information Clearinghouse for Infants with Disabilities and Life-Threatening Conditions

800-835-1043 Institute of Logopedics

800-344-5405 ABLEDATA

800-333-6293 National Center for Youth with Disabilities

800-426-2133 National Support Center for Persons with Disabilities

Disease Control
800-810-4000 Compliance Control Center

Divorce
800-733-DADS National Congress for Men and Children
800-457-6962 Mothers without Custody
800-637-7974 Parents without Partners

Down Syndrome
216-621-5858 The Baker Center
800-221-4602 National Down Syndrome Society
800-232-6372 National Down Syndrome Congress

Drug Abuse
800-729-6686 National Clearinghouse for Alcohol and Drug Information
800-662-4357 CSAT's National Drug and Alcohol Treatment Routing Service
800-667-7433 National Parents' Resource Institute for Drug Education
800-258-2766 Just Say No International

Dying, Living Wills, and Advance Directives
212-366-5540 Choice in Dying, Inc.

Dyslexia
800-222-3123 Dyslexia Society

Endometriosis
800-992-3636 Endometriosis Association

Epilepsy
800-332-1000 Epilepsy Foundation of America
800-642-0500 Epilepsy Information Service

Genital Warts
919-361-8488 American Social Health Association

Glaucoma
800-826-6693 Glaucoma Research Foundation

Government, Miscellaneous Agencies
800-358-9295 Agency for Health Care Policy and
Research Clearinghouse (AHCPR)
404-488-5080, 404-639-3311 Centers for Disease
Control and Prevention (CDC)

202-219-8148 Occupational Safety and Health Administration (OSHA)

800-669-4000 Equal Employment Opportunity Commission (EEOC)

410-597-5110 Health Care Financing Administration (HCFA)

301-443-6333 Surgeon General of the Public Health Service

301-443-2410 Food and Drug Administration (FDA)

301-443-1840 Indian Health Service

800-638-6833 Medicare Hotline

800-227-8922 CDC Nationally Sexually Transmitted Disease Hotline

800-336-4797 U.S. Public Health Service

Head/Brain Injury
800-444-6443 National Head Injury Foundation

914-883-6532 Forget-Me-Not

Headache
800-255-ACHE American Council for Headache Education

800-843-2256 National Headache Foundation

800-245-0088 New England Headache Treatment Program

Health Information

800-336-4797 National Health Information Center

Hearing/Communication Handicaps

800-424-8576 Better Hearing Institute

800-638-8255 American Speech Language Hearing Association

800-535-3323 Deafness Research Foundation

800-521-5247 Hearing Aid Helpline

800-837-8428 Vestibular Disorders Association

Heart Disease

800-242-8721, ext. 1442 Mended Hearts

214-373-6300 American Heart Association

Hemolytic Uremic Syndrome

516-673-3017 Lois Joy Galler Foundation

Hemophilia

800-424-2634 National Hemophilia Foundation

Hepatitis

800-223-0179 American Liver Foundation Hepatitis Foundation

800-891-0707 Hepatitis Foundation International

Hereditary Hemorrhagic Telangiectasia

800-448-6389 HHT Foundation

Herpes

919-361-8488 American Social Health Association

Hospice

800-658-8898 National Hospice Organization

Huntington's Disease

800-345-4372 Huntington's Disease Society

Ileitis

800-343-3637 National Foundation for Colitis and Ileitis

Immune Deficiencies

800-296-4433 Immune Deficiency Foundation

313-371-8600 AARDA

Impotence

800-843-4315 Impotence Information Center

800-867-7042 Impotency Information sponsored by Pharmacia & Upjohn, Inc.

Incontinence

800-237-4666 Simon Foundation Kidney Disease/Failure

800-622-9010 National Kidney Foundation

800-749-2257 American Association of Kidney Patients

800-638-8933 American Kidney Fund

Lead

800-424-LEAD National Lead Information Center

Liver Disease
718-987-6200 Biliary Atresia and Liver Transplant
Network
800-223-0179 American Liver Foundation

Lung Disease
800-LUNG-USA American Lung Association

Lupus
800-558-0121 Lupus Foundation
800-331-1802 American Lupus Society

Lymphedema Network
800-541-3259 National Lymphedema Network

Marfan Syndrome
800-8MARFAN National Marfan Foundation
905-826-3223 Canadian Marfan Association

Medic Alert
800-344-3226, 800-ID ALERT Medic Alert
Foundation International

Medical Transport

800-296-1217 National Patient Air Transport Hotline

Mental Health

800-447-4474 Mental Health InfoSource

207-799-6750 Creative Health Foundation

800-789-CMHS National Mental Health Services Knowledge Exchange Network

800-444-7415 National Resource Center on Homelessness and Mental Illness

800-950-6264 National Alliance for the Mentally Ill

800-783-3801 American Schizophrenia Association

Mental Retardation

817-261-6003 The Arc of the United States

Multiple Sclerosis

800-344-4867 National Multiple Sclerosis Society

Myasthenia Gravis Foundation

800-541-5454 Myasthenia Gravis Foundation

Narcolepsy

800-829-1933 Narcolepsy & Sleep Disorders

513-891-3522 Narcolepsy Network, Inc.

612-721-6321 YAWN - Young Americans With
Narcolepsy

954-452-2030 Sleep Disorders Movements, Inc.

Nurses

202-651-7000 American Nurses Association

708-966-3433 Association of Rehabilitation Nurses

800-723-0560 National Gerontological Nursing
Association

212-989-9393 National League for Nursing

312-787-6555 National Council of State Boards of
Nursing

Occupational Therapy

301-652-2682 American Occupational Therapy
Association

Organ Transplantation

818-781-1006 American Share Foundation

718-597-5619 Transplant Recipients International Org. (Manhattan Chapter)

718-987-6200 Biliary Atresia and Liver Transplant Network

800-243-6667 Organ Donor Information

Paralysis

800-225-0292 American Paralysis Association

800-962-9629 National Spinal Cord Injury Association

800-526-3456 National Spinal Cord Injury Hotline

Parkinson's Disease

800-233-2732 American Parkinson Disease Association

800-327-4545, 800-433-7022 National Parkinson Foundation

800-344-7872 Parkinson's Educational Program

Patients' Rights

617-769-5720 New England Patients' Rights Group, Inc.

Personal Hygiene
800-810-4000 Compliance Control Center

Physical Therapy
800-999-2782 American Physical Therapy Association

Pituitary Diseases
800-642-9211 Pituitary Tumor Network Association

Poison
800-962-1253 National Poison Center Network

Polio
314-534-0475 International Polio Network

Porphyria
713-266-9617 American Porphyria Foundation

Premenstrual Syndrome
800-222-4767 PMS Access

Prostatitis
309-664-6222 Prostatitis Foundation

Psoriasis
800-723-9166 National Psoriasis Foundation

Rare Diseases
203-746-6518 National Organization of Rare
Disorders

Rehabilitation
800-34-NARIC National Rehabilitation Information
Center

Restorative Medical Products
502-422-5454 Restorative Medical, Inc.

Schizophrenia
800-847-3802 American Schizophrenia Association
516-829-0091 National Alliance for Research on
Schizophrenia and Depression

Scleroderma
800-422-1113 Scleroderma Federation
800-722-4673 United Scleroderma Foundation
800-441-CURE Scleroderma Research Foundation

Scoliosis
800-673-6922 National Scoliosis Foundation, Inc.
Sexually Transmitted Diseases
800-227-8922 National STD Hotline

Sickle Cell
800-421-8453 National Association for Sickle Cell
Disease, Inc.

Social Workers
202-408-8600
National Association of Social Workers

Speech-Language-Hearing
301-897-5700 American Speech-Language-Hearing
Association

Spina Bifida

800-621-3141 Spina Bifida Association

Spinal Cord Injuries

800-962-9629 National Spinal Cord Injury Association

800-526-3456 National Spinal Cord Injury Hotline

Spinal Muscular Atrophy

800-886-1762 Families of Spinal Muscular Atrophy

Stroke

800-553-6321 Courage Stroke Network

800-787-6537 National Stroke Association

800-553-6321 American Heart Association Stroke Connection

Stuttering

800-221-2483 National Center for Stuttering

Thalassemia

800-522-7222 Thalassemia Action Group

Tourette Syndrome
800-237-0717 Tourette Syndrome Association

Wilson's Disease
800-399-0266 Wilson's Diesease Association

Women's Health
310-410-9886 Findings: The Women's Health Care Advocacy Service

JOURNALS

The following is a list of the most prominent journals on aging.

Age Page
National Institute on Aging
U.S. Department of Health and Human Services
U.S. Government Printing Office
Washington, D.C. 20402

Aging
Raven Press
1185 Avenue of the Americas
New York, NY 10036
Aging International
International Federation on Aging
380 St. Antoine Street W., Suite 3200
Montreal, Quebec, H24 3X7

American Journal of Alzheimer's Care and Releated Disorders and Research
Prime National Publishing Corporation
470 Boston Post Road
Weston, MA 02193

Clinical Gerontologist
Haworth Press
10 Alice Street
Binghampton, NY 13904-1580

Educational Gerontology
Hemisphere Publishing Corporation
1900 Frost Road, Suite 101
Briston, PA 19007
Experimental Aging Research
Taylor and Francis Publishing
1900 Frost Road, Suite 101
Briston, PA 19007

Experimental Gerontology
Pergamon Press, Inc.
660 White Plains Road
Tarrytown, NY 10591

Generations
American Society on Aging
833 Market Street, Suite 511
San Francisco, CA 94103-1824

Geriatric Nursing
Mosby-Year Book, Inc.
11830 Westline Industrial Drive
St. Louis, MO 63146

Geriatrics
Avanstar Communictions, Inc.
7500 Old Oak Boulevard
Cleveland, OH 44130

Gerontologist
Gerontological Society of America
1275 K Street N.W., Suite 350
Washington, D.C. 20005-4006
Gerontology and Geriatrics Education
Haworth Press, Inc.
10 Alice Street
Binghamton, NY 13904

**International Journal of Aging and Human
Development**
Baywood Publishing Co., Inc.
26 Austin Avenue, Box 337
Amityville, NY 11701

Journal of Aging and Health
Sage Publications
2455 Telber Road
Newsbury Park, CA 91320

Journal of Aging and Social Policy
Haworth Press, Inc.
10 Alice Street
Binghamton, NY 13904

Journal of the American Geriatrics Society
Williams and Wilkins
428 East Preston Street
Baltimore, MD 21202-3993
Journal of Geriatric Psychiatry
International Universities Press, Inc.
59 Boston Road
Madison, CT 06443-1542

Journal of Gerontological Nursing
Slack, Inc.
6900 Grove road
Thorofare, NJ 08086-9447

Journal of Long-Term Care Administration
American College of Health Care Administrators
325 S. Patrick Avenue
Alexandria, VA 22314

Journal of Nutrition for the Elderly
Haworth Press, Inc.
10 Alice Street
Binghamton, NY 13904

Perspective on Aging
National Council on the Aging
409 3rd Street S.W.
Washington, D.C. 20024

STATE AGENCIES ON AGING

Alabama
Commission on Aging
770 Washington Ave., Suite 470
Montgomery, AL 36130-1851
(800) 243-5463 or (205) 242-5743

Alaska
Older Alaskans Commission
PO Box 110209
Juneau, AK 99811
(907) 465-3250

American Samoa
Territorial Administration on Aging
Government of American Samoa
Pago Pago, AS 96799
(684) 633-1252

Arizona

Dept. of Economic Security

Aging & Adult Administration

1789 W. Jefferson St.

Phoenix, AZ 85007

(602) 542-4446

Arkansas

Division of Aging and Adult Services

1417 Donaghey Plaza South

PO Box 1437/Slot 1412

Little Rock, AR 72203-1437

(501) 682-2441 or (800) 852-5494

California

Department of Aging

1600 K Street

Sacramento, CA 95814

(916) 322-3887

Colorado
Aging and Adult Services
Dept. of Social Services
1575 Sherman St., 4th Floor
Denver, CO 80203-1714
(303) 866-3851

Connecticut
Department on Aging
175 Main Street
Hartford, CT 06106
(800) 443-9946 or (203) 566-7772

Delaware
Division of Aging
Department of Health & Social Services
1901 N. DuPont Highway
2nd Floor Annex, Admin. Bldg.
New Castle, DE 19720
(302) 577-4791

District of Columbia
Office on Aging
1424 K Street, NW
2nd Floor
Washington, DC 20005
(202) 724-5626

Florida
Department of Elder Affairs
1317 Winewood Boulevard
Building 1, Room 317
Tallahassee, FL 32301
(904) 922-5297

Georgia
Office of Aging
Department of Human Resources
878 Peachtree St., NE, Room 632
Atlanta, GA 30309
(404) 894-5333

Guam
Division of Senior Citizens
Department of Public
Health and Social Services
PO Box 2816
Agana, Guam 96910
(671) 734-4361

Hawaii
Department of Commerce
Executive Office on Aging and Consumer Affairs
335 Merchant Street, Room 241
Honolulu, HI 96813
(808) 586-0100

Idaho
Office on Aging
Statehouse, Room 108
Boise, ID 83720
(208) 334-3833

Illinois

Department on Aging
421 E. Capitol Avenue
Springfield, IL 62701
(217) 785-3356

Indiana

Division of Aging and Home Services
402 W. Washington Street
PO Box 7083
Indianapolis, IN 46207-7083
(317) 232-7020 or (800) 545-7763

Iowa

Department of Elder Affairs
Jewett Building., Suite 236
914 Grand Avenue
Des Moines, IA 50319
(515) 281-5187

Kansas
Department on Aging
122-S Docking
State Office Building
915 SW Harrison
Topeka, KS 66612-1500
(913) 296-4986

Kentucky
Division of Aging Services
Cabinet for Human Resources
275 E. Main Street
Frankfort, KY 40621
(502) 564-6930

Louisiana
Governor's Office of Elderly Affairs
4550 N. Boulevard
PO Box 80374
Baton Rouge, LA 70898-0374
(504) 925-1700

CLINICAL
REFERRALS

Maine
Bureau of Elder and Adult Services
State House, Station 11
Augusta, ME 04333
(207) 624-5335

Maryland
Office on Aging
301 W. Preston Street, Room 1004
Baltimore, MD 21201
(410) 225-1100

Massachusetts
Executive Office of Elder Affairs
1 Ashburton Place, 5th Floor
Boston, MA 02108
(800) 882-2003 or (617) 727-7750

Michigan
Office of Services to the Aging
611 W. Ottawa Street
PO Box 30026
Lansing, MI 48909
(517) 373-8230

Minnesota
Board on Aging
Human Services Building, 4th Floor
444 Lafayette Road
St. Paul, MN 55155-3843
(612) 296-2770

Mississippi
Division of Aging and Adult Services
455 N. Lamar Street
Jackson, MS 39202
(800) 345-6347 or (601) 359-6770

Missouri
Division of Aging
Dept. of Social Services
PO Box 1337
615 Howerton Court
Jefferson City, MO 65102-1337
(314) 751-3082

Montana

Governor's Office on Aging
State Capitol Building, Room 219
Helena, MT 59620
(800) 332-2272 or (406) 444-3111

Nebraska

Department on Aging
State Office Building
301 Centennial Mall South
Lincoln, NE 68509-5044
(402) 471-2306

Nevada

Department of Human Resources
Division for Aging Services
340 N. 11th Street, Suite 114
Las Vegas, NV 89101
(702) 486-3545

New Hampshire
Dept. of Health & Human Services
Division of Elderly & Adult Services
State Office Park S.
115 Pleasant Street, Annex Bldg. #1
Concord, NH 03301
(603) 271-4680

New Jersey
Dept. of Community Affairs
Division on Aging
101 S. Broad and Front Streets
CN807
Trenton, NJ 08625-0807
(800) 792-8820 or (609) 984-3951

New Mexico
State Agency on Aging
La Villa Rivera Bldg.
224 E. Palace Ave.
Santa Fe, NM 87501
(800) 432-2080 or (505) 827-7640

New York
State Office for the Aging
Two Empire State Plaza
Albany, NY 12223-0001
(800) 342-9871 or (518) 474-5731

North Carolina
Division of Aging
693 Palmer Drive, Caller Box 29531
Raleigh, NC 27626-0531
(919) 733-3983

North Dakota
Department of Human Services
Aging Services Division
PO Box 7070
Bismarck, ND 58507-7070
(701) 224-2577

Ohio
Department of Aging
50 W. Broad Street, 8th Floor
Columbus, OH 43266-0501
(614) 466-1221

Oklahoma
Department of Human Services
Aging Services Division
312 NE 28th Street
Oklahoma City, OK 73125
(405) 521-2327

Oregon
Dept. of Human Resources
Senior and Disabled Services Division
500 Summer Street, NE, 2nd Floor
Salem, OR 97310-1015
(800) 282-8096 or (503) 378-4728

Pennsylvania
Department of Aging
231 State Street
Barto Building
Harrisburg, PA 17101
(717) 783-1550

Puerto Rico
Governor's Office for Elderly Affairs
Gericulture Commission
PO Box 11398
Santurce, PR 00910
(809) 722-2429

Rhode Island
Department of Elderly Affairs
160 Pine Street
Providence, RI 02903
(401) 277-2858

South Carolina
Commission on Aging
400 Arbor Lake Drive, Suite B-500
Columbia, SC 29223
(803) 735-0210

South Dakota
Office of Adult Services and Aging
700 Governors Drive
Pierre, SD 57501-2291
(605) 773-3656

Tennessee
Commission on Aging
706 Church Street, Office Suite 201
Nashville, TN 37243
(615) 741-2056

CLINICAL
REFERRALS

Texas

Department on Aging

PO Box 12786

Austin, TX 78711

(512) 444-2727

Utah

Division of Aging & Adult Services

120 North 200 West, Room 401

PO Box 45500

Salt Lake City, UT 84103

(801) 538-3910

Vermont

Department of Aging and Disabilities

Waterbury Complex

103 S. Main Street

Waterbury, VT 05671-2301

(802) 241-2400

Virginia
Department for the Aging
700 Centre, 10th Floor
700 E. Franklin Street
Richmond, VA 23219-2327
(800) 552-4464 or (804) 225-2271

Virgin Islands
Senior Citizens Affairs Division
19 Estate Diamond
Fredericksted
St. Croix, VI 00840
(809) 774-0930

Washington
Aging & Adult Services Administration
PO Box 40505
Department of Social
Olympia, WA 98504-5050
(206) 586-3768

West Virginia
Commission on Aging
State Capitol Complex
Holly Grove
1900 Kanawha Blvd. East
Charleston, WV
25305-0160 or (304) 558-3317

Wisconsin
Bureau on Aging
Dept. of Health and Social Services
PO Box 7851
One W. Wilson Street
Madison, WI 53707-7851
(608) 266-2536

Wyoming
Commission on Aging
Hathaway Building
2300 Capitol Ave., Room 139
Cheyenne, WY 82002
(800) 442-2766 or (307) 777-7986

FEDERAL AGENCIES

Agency for Health Care Policy and Research
Division of Communications
2101 E. Jefferson St.
Rockville, MD 20852
(301) 594-1364

Agency for Toxic Substances and Disease Registry
1600 Clifton Road NE
Mail Stop E28
Atlanta, GA 30333
(404) 639-0700

Alcohol, Drug Abuse and Mental Health
Administration
Parklawn Building
5600 Fishers Lane
Rockville, Maryland 20857
(301) 443-2403

Centers for Disease Control
2000 Building 1
1600 Clifton Rd., NE
Atlanta, GA 30333
(404) 639-3311

Equal Employment Opportunity Commission
1801 L. St., NW
Washington, DC 20510
(800) 669-4000

Food and Drug Administration
Parklawn Building
5600 Fishers Lane
Rockville, MD 20857
(301) 443-2410

Health Care Financing Administration
Security Office Park Building, Room 1A11
7008 Security Blvd.
Baltimore, MD 21207
(410) 597-5110

Health Resources and Services Administration
Division of Nursing
5600 Fishers Lane, Room 9-35
Rockville, MD 20857
(301) 443-5786

Indian Health Service
12300 Twinbrook Parkway
Twinbrook Metro Plaza, Suite 100
Rockville, MD 20852
(301) 443-1840

National Institute on Alcohol Abuse and Alcoholism
16-05 Parklawn Building
5600 Fishers Lane
Rockville, Maryland 20857
(301) 443-3885

National Institute on Drug Abuse
10-05 Parklawn Building
5600 Fishers Lane
Rockville, Maryland 20857
(301) 443-6480

National Institutes of Health
9000 Rockville Pike
Bethesda, Maryland 20892
(301) 496-4000

National Institute on Mental Health
17-105 Parklawn Building
5600 Fishers Lane
Rockville, Maryland 20857
(301) 443-3673

National Library of Medicine Office of Inquiries and
Publications Management
M121 Building 38
8600 Rockville Pike
Bethesda, Maryland 20894
(301) 443-3673

Occupational Safety and Health Administration
(OSHA)
Department of Labor
200 Constitution Avenue NW
N-36-47
Washington, D.C. 20010
(202) 523-8148

Surgeon General of the Public Health Service
5600 Fishers Lane, Room 9-36
Rockville, MD 20857
(301) 443-6333

Other Agencies

Joint Commission on Accreditation of Healthcare
Organizations
1 Renaissance Blvd.
Oakbrook Terrace, IL 60181
(630) 792-5000
(630) 792-5005 (fax)

STATE BOARDS OF NURSING
CONTACT INFORMATION

National Council of State Boards of Nursing, Inc.
676 North St. Clair; Suite 550
Chicago, IL 60611
(312) 787-6555
http://www.ncsbn.org

Alabama Board of Nursing
P.O. Box 303900
Montgomery, AL 36130
Phone: (334) 242-4060
FAX: (334) 242-4360
Executive Director: Judi Crume, Executive Officer

Alaska Board of Nursing
Dept. of Comm. & Econ. Development
Div. of Occupational Licensing
3601 C Street, Suite 722
Anchorage, AK 99503
Phone: (907) 269-8161FAX: (907) 269-8156
Executive Director: Dorothy Fulton, Executive
Director

American Samoa Health Services
Regulatory Board
LBJ Tropical Medical Center
Pago Pago, AS 96799
Phone: (684) 633-1222
FAX: (684) 633-1869
Executive Director: Marie Ma'o, Director, Nursing Services

Arizona State Board of Nursing
1651 E. Morten Avenue, Suite 150
Phoenix, AZ 85020
Phone: (602) 255-5092
FAX: (602) 255-5130
http://www.state.az.us/bn/welcome.html
Executive Director: Joey Ridenour, Executive Director

Arkansas State Board of Nursing
University Tower Building
1123 S. University, Suite 800
Little Rock, AR 72204
Phone: (501) 686-2700
FAX: (501) 686-2714
Executive Director: Faith Fields, Executive Director

California Board of Registered Nursing
P.O. Box 944210
Sacramento, CA 94244
Phone: (916) 322-3350
FAX: (916) 327-4402
Executive Director: Ruth Ann Terry, Executive Officer

California Board of Vocational Nurse
and Psychiatric Technician Examiners
2535 Capitol Oaks Drive, Suite 205
Sacramento, CA 95833
Phone: (916) 263-7800
FAX: (916) 263-7859
Executive Director: Teresa Bello-Jones, Executive
Officer

Colorado Board of Nursing
1560 Broadway, Suite 670
Denver, CO 80202
Phone: (303) 894-2430
FAX: (303) 894-2821
Executive Director: Karen Brumley, Program
Administrator

Connecticut Board of Examiners for Nursing
Division of Health Systems Regulation
410 Capitol Avenue, MS# 12HSR
Hartford, CT 06134
Phone: (860) 509-7624
FAX: (860) 509-7286
Executive Director: Wendy Furniss, Health Services
Supervisor, Certification

Delaware Board of Nursing
Cannon Building, Suite 203
P.O. Box 1401
Dover, DE 19903
Phone: (302) 739-4522
FAX: (302) 739-2711
Executive Director: Iva Boardman, Executive Director

District of Columbia Board of Nursing
614 H. Street, N.W.
Washington, DC 20001
Phone: (202) 727-7468
FAX: (202) 727-7662
Executive Director: Barbara Hagans, Contact Person

Florida Board of Nursing
4080 Woodcock Drive, Suite 202
Jacksonville, FL 32207
Phone: (904) 858-6940
FAX: (904) 858-6964
Executive Director: Marilyn Bloss, Executive Director

Georgia State Board of Licensed
Practical Nurses
166 Pryor Street, S.W.
Atlanta, GA 30303
Phone: (404) 656-3921
FAX: (404) 651-9532
Executive Director: Patricia Swann, Executive
Director

Georgia Board of Nursing
166 Pryor Street, S.W.
Atlanta, GA 30303
Phone: (404) 656-3943
FAX: (404) 657-7489
Executive Director: Shirley Camp, Executive Director

Guam Board of Nurse Examiners
P.O. Box 2816
Agana, GU 96910
Phone: (671) 475-0251
FAX: (671) 477-4733
Executive Director: Teofila Cruz, Nurse Examiner
Administrator

Hawaii Board of Nursing
P.O. Box 3469
Honolulu, HI 96801
Phone: (808) 586-2695
FAX: (808) 586-2689
Executive Director: Kathleen Yokouchi, Executive
Officer

Idaho Board of Nursing
P.O. Box 83720
Boise, ID 83720
Phone: (208) 334-3110
FAX: (208) 334-3262
Executive Director: Sandra Evans, Executive Director

Illinois Department of Professional Regulation
James R. Thompson Center
100 West Randolph, Suite 9-300
Chicago, IL 60601
Phone: (312) 814-2715
FAX: (312) 814-3145
http://www.state.il.us/dr
Executive Director: Jacqueline Waggoner, Nursing
Act Coordinator

Indiana State Board of Nursing
Health Professions Bureau
402 W. Washington Street, Suite 041
Indianapolis, IN 46204
Phone: (317) 232-2960
FAX: (317) 233-4236
Executive Director: Laura Langford, Executive
Director

Iowa Board of Nursing
State Capitol Complex
1223 East Court Avenue
Des Moines, IA 50319
Phone: (515) 281-3255
FAX: (515) 281-4825
Executive Director: Lorinda Inman, Executive
Director

Kansas State Board of Nursing
Landon State Office Building
900 S.W. Jackson, Suite 551-S
Topeka, KS 66612
Phone: (913) 296-4929
FAX: (913) 296-3929
http://www.ink.org/public/ksbn
Executive Director: Patsy Johnson, Executive
Administrator

Kentucky Board of Nursing
312 Whittington Parkway, Suite 300
Louisville, KY 40222
Phone: (502) 329-7006
FAX: (502) 329-7011
Executive Director: Sharon Weisenbeck, Executive
Director

Louisiana State Board of Practical
Nurse Examiners
3421 N. Causeway Boulevard, Suite 203
Metairie, LA 70002
Phone: (504) 838-5791
FAX: (504) 838-5279
Executive Director: Terry DeMarcay, Executive
Director

Louisiana State Board of Nursing
3510 N. Causeway Boulevard, Suite 501
Metairie, LA 70002
Phone: (504) 838-5332
FAX: (504) 838-5349
Executive Director: Barbara Morvant, Executive
Director

Maine State Board of Nursing
24 Stone Street
State House Station #158
Augusta, ME 04333
Phone: (207) 287-1133
FAX: (207) 287-1149
Executive Director: Jean Caron, Executive Director

Maryland Board of Nursing
4140 Patterson Avenue
Baltimore, MD 21215
Phone: (410) 764-5124
FAX: (410) 358-3530
Executive Director: Donna Dorsey, Executive Director

Massachusetts Board of Registration in Nursing
Leverett Saltonstall Building
100 Cambridge Street, Room 1519
Boston, MA 02202
Phone: (617) 727-9961
FAX: (617) 727-2197
Executive Director: Theresa Bonanno, Executive
Director

State of Michigan
CIS/Office of Health Services
Ottawa Towers North
611 W. Ottawa, 4th Floor
Lansing, MI 48933
Phone: (517) 373-9102
FAX: (517) 373-2179
Executive Director: Carol Johnson, Licensing
Administrator (Board Support
Section)

Minnesota Board of Nursing
2829 University Avenue SE
Suite 500
Minneapolis, MN 55414
Phone: (612) 617-2270
FAX: (612) 617-2190
Executive Director: Joyce Schowalter, Executive
Director

Mississippi Board of Nursing
239 N. Lamar Street, Suite 401
Jackson, MS 39201
Phone: (601) 359-6170
FAX: (601) 359-6185
Executive Director: Marcia Rachel, Executive
Director

Missouri State Board of Nursing
P.O. Box 656
Jefferson City, MO 65102
Phone: (573) 751-0681
FAX: (573) 751-0075
http://www.ecodev.state.mo.us/pr/nursing
Executive Director: Florence Stillman, Executive
Director

Montana State Board of Nursing
111 North Jackson
P.O. Box 200513
Helena, MT 59620
Phone: (406) 444-2071
FAX: (406) 444-7759
Executive Director: Dianne Wickham, Executive
Director
Professional and Occupational Licensure Division

Nebraska Department of Health
P.O. Box 94986
Lincoln, NE 68509
Phone: (402) 471-4376
FAX: (402) 471-3577
Executive Director: Charlene Kelly, Section
Administrator

Nevada State Board of Nursing
1755 East Plumb Lane
Suite 260
Reno, NV 89502
Phone: (702) 786-2778
FAX: (702) 322-6993
Executive Director: Kathy Apple, Executive Director

New Hampshire Board of Nursing
Health & Welfare Building
6 Hazen Drive
Concord, NH 03301
Phone: (603) 271-2323
FAX: (603) 271-6605
Executive Director: Doris Nuttelman, Executive
Director

New Jersey Board of Nursing
P.O. Box 45010
Newark, NJ 07101
Phone: (201) 504-6586
FAX: (201) 648-3481
Executive Director: Margaret Howard, Field
Representative

New Mexico Board of Nursing
4206 Louisiana Boulevard, NE
Suite A
Albuquerque, NM 87109
Phone: (505) 841-8340
FAX: (505) 841-8347
Executive Director: Nancy Twigg, Executive Director

New York State Board of Nursing
State Education Department
Cultural Education Center, Room 3023
Albany, NY 12230
Phone: (518) 474-3843
FAX: (518) 473-0578
Executive Director: Milene Sower, Executive Secretary

Commonwealth Board of Nurse Examiners
Public Health Center
P.O. Box 1458
Saipan, MP 96950
Phone: (670) 234-8950
FAX: (670) 234-8930
Executive Director: Elizabeth Torres-Untalan,
Chairperson

North Carolina Board of Nursing
3724 National Drive
Raleigh, NC 27602
Phone: (919) 782-3211
FAX: (919) 781-9461
Executive Director: Carol Osman, Executive Director

North Dakota Board of Nursing
919 South 7th Street, Suite 504
Bismarck, ND 58504
Phone: (701) 328-9777
FAX: (701) 328-9785
Executive Director: Ida Rigley, Executive Director

Ohio Board of Nursing
77 South High Street, 17th Floor
Columbus, OH 43266
Phone: (614) 466-3947
FAX: (614) 466-0388
http://www.state.oh.us/nur
Executive Director: Dorothy Fiorino, Executive
Director

Oklahoma Board of Nursing
2915 N. Classen Boulevard, Suite 524
Oklahoma City, OK 73106
Phone: (405) 525-2076
FAX: (405) 521-6089
Executive Director: Sulinda Moffett, Executive
Director

Oregon State Board of Nursing
800 NE Oregon Street, Box 25
Suite 465
Portland, OR 97232
Phone: (503) 731-4745
FAX: (503) 731-4755
Executive Director: Joan Bouchard, Executive
Director

Pennsylvania State Board of Nursing
P.O. Box 2649
Harrisburg, PA 17105
Phone: (717) 783-7142
FAX: (717) 783-0822
Executive Director: Miriam Limo, Executive Secretary

Commonwealth of Puerto Rico
Board of Nurse Examiners
Call Box 10200
Santurce, PR 00908
Phone: (787) 725-8161
FAX: (787) 725-7903
Executive Director: Beverly Dabula, Executive
Director

Rhode Island Board of Nurse
Registration and Nursing Education
Cannon Health Building
Three Capitol Hill, Room 104
Providence, RI 02908
Phone: (401) 277-2827
FAX: (401) 277-1272
Executive Director: Carol Lietar, Executive Officer

South Carolina State Board of Nursing
220 Executive Center Drive, Suite 220
Columbia, SC 29210
Phone: (803) 731-1648
FAX: (803) 731-1647
Executive Director: Barbara Kellogg, Program Nurse
Consultant

South Dakota Board of Nursing
3307 South Lincoln Avenue
Sioux Falls, SD 57105
Phone: (605) 367-5940
FAX: (605) 367-5945
Executive Director: Diana Vander Woude, Executive
Secretary

Tennessee State Board of Nursing
426 Fifth Avenue North
1st Floor - Cordell Hull Building
Nashville, TN 37247
Phone: (615) 532-5166
FAX: (615) 741-7899
Executive Director: Elizabeth Lund, Executive Director

Texas Board of Nurse Examiners
P.O. Box 140466
Austin, TX 78714
Phone: (512) 305-7400
FAX: (512) 305-7401
http://www.bne.state.tx.us
Executive Director: Katherine Thomas, Executive Director

Texas Board of Vocational Nurse Examiners
William P. Hobby Building, Tower 3
333 Guadalupe Street, Suite 3-400
Austin, TX 78701
Phone: (512) 305-8100
FAX: (512) 305-8101
http://www.state.tx.us/agency/511.html
Executive Director: Marjorie Bronk, Executive
Director

Utah State Board of Nursing
Division of Occupational and Professional Licensing
P.O. Box 45805
Salt Lake City, UT 84145
Phone: (801) 530-6628
FAX: (801) 530-6511
http://www.commerce.state.ut.us/web/commerce/DO
PL/dopl1.htm
Executive Director: Laura Poe, Executive
Administrator

Vermont State Board of Nursing
109 State Street
Montpelier, VT 05609
Phone: (802) 828-2396
FAX: (802) 828-2484
Executive Director: Anita Ristau, Executive Director

Virgin Islands Board of Nurse Licensure
P.O. Box 4247
Veterans Drive Station
St. Thomas, VI 00803
Phone: (809) 776-7397
FAX: (809) 777-4003
Executive Director: Winifred Garfield, Executive
Secretary

Virginia Board of Nursing
6606 W. Broad Street, 4th Floor
Richmond, VA 23230
Phone: (804) 662-9909
FAX: (804) 662-9943
http://www.dhp.state.va.us
Executive Director: Nancy Durrett, Executive
Director

Washington State Nursing Care Quality
Assurance Commission
Department of Health
P.O. Box 47864
Olympia, WA 98504
Phone: (360) 753-2686
FAX: (360) 586-5935
Executive Director: Patty Hayes, Executive Director

West Virginia State Board
of Examiners for Practical Nurses
101 Dee Drive
Charleston, WV 25311
Phone: (304) 558-3572
FAX: (304) 558-4367
Executive Director: Nancy Wilson, Executive
Secretary

West Virginia Board of Examiners
for Registered Professional Nurses
101 Dee Drive
Charleston, WV 25311
Phone: (304) 558-3596
FAX: (304) 558-3666
Executive Director: Laura Skidmore Rhodes,
Executive Secretary

Wisconsin Department of Regulation
and Licensing
1400 E. Washington Avenue
P.O. Box 8935
Madison, WI 53708
Phone: (608) 266-2112
FAX: (608) 267-0644
http://www.state.wi.us
Executive Director: Thomas Neumann,
Administrative Officer

Wyoming State Board of Nursing
2020 Carey Avenue, Suite 110
Cheyenne, WY 82002
Phone: (307) 777-7601
FAX: (307) 777-3519
Executive Director: Toma Nisbet, Executive Director

INTERNET LIST OF NURSING BOARDS

National Council of State Boards of Nursing, Inc.
http://www.ncsbn.org

Arizona State Board of Nursing
http://www.state.az.us/bn/welcome.html

Arkansas State Board of Nursing
http://www.state.ar.us/nurse/abn1.html

Illinois Department of Registration and Education
http://www.state.il.us/dpr

Kansas State Board of Nursing
http://www.ink.org/public/ksbn

Maryland Board of Nursing
http://www.mop.md.gov/mbn/

Missouri State Board of Nursing
http://www.ecodev.state.mo.us/pr/nursing

New York info for licensure
http://www.nysed.gov

Ohio Board of Nursing
http://www.state.oh.us/nur

Texas Board of Nurse Examiners
http://www.bne.state.tx.us

Texas Board of Vocational Nurse Examiners
http://www.state.tx.us/agency/511.html

Utah State Board of Nursing
http://www.commerce.state.ut.us/web/commerce/DO
PL/dopl1.htm

Vermont Board of Nursing
http://www.sec.state.vt.us/opr/rules/nursing/nursedex.
htm

Virginia Board of Nursing
http://www.dhp.state.va.us

Wisconsin Department of Regulation and Licensing
http://www.state.wi.us

INDEX

INDEX

Other Publications From
Skidmore-Roth Publishing, Inc.

	CODE	ISBN #	PRICE	QTY
INSTANT INSTRUCTOR SERIES				
AIDS/HIV	ADIN01	1-56930-010-0	$ 16.95	
C.C.U.	CCINC1	1-56930-022-4	$ 16.95	
Diabetes	DBII01	1-56930-041-0	$ 16.95	
Geriatric	GRN01	0-944132-68-5	$ 16.95	
Hemodialysis	DLIN01	1-56930-020-8	$ 16.95	
I.C.U.	ICUI01	1-56930-021-6	$ 16.95	
IV	IVII01	1-56930-043-7	$ 16.95	
Lab	LBIN01	0-944132-70-7	$ 16.95	
Obstetric	OBIN01	0-944132-67-7	$ 16.95	
Oncology	ONIN01	1-56930-023-2	$ 16.95	
Pediatric	PDIN01	0-944132-66-9	$ 16.95	
Psychiatric	PSY101	0-944132-69-3	$ 16.95	
NURSING CARE PLANS SERIES				
AIDS/HIV	ADSC01	0-56930-000-3	$ 36.95	
Critical Care	CNCP01	1-56930-035-6	$ 36.95	
Geriatric (2nd ed.)	GNCP02	1-56930-052-6	$ 36.95	
Oncology	ONCP01	1-56930-004-6	$ 36.95	
Pediatric (2nd ed.)	PNOP02	1-56930-057-7	$ 38.95	
SURVIVAL SERIES				
	GSGD01	1-56930-061-5	$ 29.95	
Nurse's Survival Guide (2nd ed.)	NSGD02	0-944132-75-8	$ 29.95	
Obstetric Survival	OBSG01	0-944132-94-4	$ 29.95	
Pediatric Survival Guide	PNGD01	1-56930-018-6	$ 29.95	
RN NCLEX REVIEW SERIES				
Concepts of Medical Surgical Nursing	NMS01	0-944132-85-5	$ 21.95	
Concepts of Obstetric Nursing	NOB01	0-944132-86-3	$ 21.95	
Concepts of Psychiatric Nursing	NPSY01	0-944132-83-9	$ 21.95	
PN/VN Review Cards (2nd ed.)	PNRC02	1-56930-008-9	$ 29.95	
RN Review Cards (2nd ed.)	RNRC02	0-944132-82-0	$ 29.95	

Other Publications From
Skidmore-Roth Publishing, Inc.

	CODE	ISBN #	PRICE	QTY
NURSING/OTHER				
Body in Brief (3rd ed.)	BBRF03	1-56930-055-0	$ 35.95	
Diagnostic and Lab Cards (2nd ed.)	DLC02	0-944132-77-4	$ 27.95	
Drug Comparison Handbook (2nd ed.)	DRUG02	1-56930-16-x	$ 35.95	
Essential Laboratory Mathematics	ELM01	1-56930-056-9	$ 29.95	
Geriatric Long-Term Procedures & Treatments	GLTP01	0-944132-97-9	$ 34.95	
Geriatric Nutrition and Diet (2nd ed.)	NUT02	1-56930-045-3	$ 19.95	
Long Term Care, A Skills Handbook (2nd ed.)	HLTC02	1-56930-058-5	$ 23.95	
Handbook for Nurse Assistants (2nd ed.)	HNA02	1-56930-059-3	$ 23.95	
I.C.U. Quick Reference	ICQU01	1-56930-003-8	$ 32.95	
Infection Control	INFC01	1-56930-051-8	$ 99.95	
Nursing Diagnosis Cards (2nd ed.)	NDC02	1-56930-060-7	$ 29.95	
Nurse's Trivia Calendar, 1998	NTC98	1-56930-073-9	$ 11.95	
OBRA (2nd ed.)	OBRA02	1-56930-046-1	$ 99.95	
OSHA Book (2nd ed.)	OSHA02	1-56930-069-0	$ 119.95	
Procedure Cards (3rd ed.)	PCCU03	1-56930-054-2	$ 24.95	
Pharmacy Tech	PHAR01	1-56930-005-4	$ 25.95	
Spanish for Medical Personnel	SPAN01	1-56930-001-1	$ 21.95	
Staff Develop for the Psych Nurse	STDEV0	0-944132-78-2	$ 59.95	
OUTLINE SERIES				
Diabetes Outline	DB)L01	1-56930-031-3	$ 23.95	
Fundamentals of Nursing Outline	FUND01	1-56930-029-1	$ 23.95	
Geriatric Outline	GER01	0-944132-90-1	$ 23.95	
Hemodynamic Monitoring Outline	HDMO01	1-56930-034-8	$ 23.95	
High Acuity Outline	HATO01	1-56930-028-3	$ 23.95	
Medical-Surgical Nursing Outline (2nd ed.)	MSN02	1-56930-068-2	$ 23.95	
Obstetric Nursing Outline (2nd ed.)	OBS02	1-56930-070-4	$ 23.95	
Pediatric Nursing Outline	PN01	0-944132-89-8	$ 23.95	

Name _____

Address _____

City _____

State _____ Zip _____

Phone ( ) _____

    ❏ VISA   ❏ MasterCard   ❏ American Express

    ❏ Check/Money Order

Card # _____ Expiration Date _____

Signature (required) _____

Prices subject to change. Please add $6.95 each for postage and handling. Include your local sales tax.

Mail or Fax your order to:

SKIDMORE-ROTH PUBLISHING, INC.
2620 S. Parker Road, Suite 147
Aurora, Colorado 80014
1 (800) 825-3150 – FAX (303) 306-1460

or

Visit our website at: http://www.skidmore-roth.com